the cardiologist's wife's

CHOCOLATE TOO! *DIET*

No Sugar, No Fat & Luscious

Joyce and Robert G. Schneider, M.D.

Copyright © 2007 Joyce and Robert G. Schneider, M.D.
All rights reserved.

ISBN: 1-4196-7363-7
ISBN-13: 978-1419673634

Visit www.booksurge.com to order additional copies.

This book is dedicated to Dieters everywhere,
to your persistence, courage, and good health.

• • •

Robert G. Schneider, M.D. has practiced internal medicine and clinical cardiology for more than 30 years, has served as Chief of Medicine in the Strategic Air Command, and is a Senior Attending Physician Emeritus, Departments of Medicine and Cardiology of Norwalk Hospital, Norwalk, CT. He is also a Consultant for the Connecticut Department of Public Health, and a federal and state designated First Responder. He has authored ground-breaking articles for the American Heart Journal and the New York State Journal of Medicine, as well as written the books WHEN TO SAY NO TO SURGERY and CANCER PREVENTION MADE EASY for the general public.

Joyce Schneider loves to cook and write. She has spent twenty-five years perfecting Heart Smart Cooking, getting it better with each new finding in Nutrition and Cardiology. In addition she has written DARKNESS FALLS and STRYKER'S CHILDREN, both thrillers, and FLORA TRISTAN, a biography for young adults.

CONTENTS

PART ONE

Most Recent Update in Nutrition and Cardiology

Unsweetened cocoa: blockbuster drug.......................................3
Healthy New Food Products = new ways to prepare food..........4
Anytime Brownies and Blondies™:
    No sugar, No fat, & 19 g. protein per serving...........................5
Trans Fats: Still in our Food...6
"Good carbs, bad carbs?" 6
Awful Diets..7
"Speed Up Your Metabolism?" 15
Amazing Facts About Your Heart and Blood Sugar 17
Fructose, The New Danger..27
Artificial Sweeteners 28
Only the Rich Used to be Fed-Too-Wells 30
Younger Plaque is More Dangerous 32
Statin Drugs, Belly Bands, & Hoodia......................................33
The Nazi Occupation of Norway: Uncomfortable Facts 36
Exercise 45

PART TWO

Food Lists, Meal Plans, & Recipes

New Food Products for Diet and Health..................................57
Daily Meal Plans 65

Recipes: Breakfasts, Lunches, & Snacks...................................87
          Entrees 102
          Desserts and Healthy Sweets...................................122

PART THREE

A Physician Explains Tests, Drugs, & Doctor-Speak..............135
Body Mass Index 145

PART FOUR

Hidden Sugar in your Old Diet Recipes 149
How to Replace with New Food Products 154
Index...173

PART ONE
Update in Nutrition and Cardiology

NOTHING TASTES AS GOOD
AS BEING THIN FEELS

CHAPTER ONE
Losing Weight Has Never Been Easier

Here at last is a diet you can stick to for life. With great meals and snacks, but a diet whose engine – what will keep you feeling good -- is chocolate. The hug drug, the feel-better drug. Dieting or keeping those hard-won pounds off is so hard without the chocolate we crave ...so what if you could diet *and* have chocolate?

Unsweetened cocoa, that is, and amazing things you can do now with it and artificial sweeteners. In fact, it's required in this astonishing new diet designed by a noted cardiologist with 30 years' clinical experience and his wife, an inventive Heart-Smart Cook. ("Eat your chocolate!" ☺) **Unsweetened cocoa is a blockbuster drug.** It helps us immeasurably, physically and emotionally. Would it be overstating to call it a fountain of youth?

Imagine a newly discovered drug that could: hyper-boost your antioxidant levels; diminish the aging process; prevent viruses (flu, common cold); lower your blood pressure; help prevent cancer, strokes and heart attacks; AND produce that endorphinny good feeling (relaxing artery walls, increasing a sense of optimism *like a mood altering drug*) that helps you stick to a diet, lose the weight which overwhelmingly causes those diseases.

Researchers & drug companies have spent decades & billions searching, little suspecting that...

...it was in unsweetened cocoa all along.

A dream come true if you're just trying to lose weight. A godsend if you're on Lipitor and Lopressor -- which, continue taking, if prescribed -- and your doctor has told you to lose...fifty pounds? Sixty? Nooo! It's too hard! All the other diets failed, right??

Right. Because, even if they preached the vital stick-to-lean-chicken-fish-and-veggies credo...you still starved, got bored, impatient, and too often gave in to your cravings.

But a diet that includes feel-better, make-in-seconds gooey chocolate? Good-bye boredom, cravings, and diet stress! Thank goodness for soy products that act like flour, safe[1] artificial sweeteners, fat-free cooking sprays, and egg replacers to save you from artery-clogging cholesterol. But how to put all these together? Cook, bake, and prepare *all* food in a whole new way? Surprise: even with this diet's shrimp scampi or no-yolks quiche or gorgeous pasta, you may start seeing the meal as the cover act and dessert as the headliner!

Two things have come together: alarm over our national epidemic of obesity, heart disease, & diabetes; and food manufacturers' response to the crisis with delicious but **healthy New Food Products**.

(Google "health benefits of unsweetened cocoa" -- or simply, "flavanols" – the most multi-tasking of all antioxidants; a superfood, with wellness powers vastly higher than green tea, blueberries, broccoli, all of them.)

And...call us the Cook and the Cardiologist. I'm the Cook, coached for years by my husband on every new finding in Nutrition and Cardiology, with frequent protests of "I WANT FUDGE!" Then I heard about the cocoa findings, got excited, combined cocoa

1   Except for fructose. See p. 27.

& other New Food Products with our regular, decades-old Keep UsThin Diet that's worked *despite really wicked binges,* & created "hybrid recipes" that are fun. I'll teach you **new ways to prepare food** that will get you thin and healthy permanently, with greater ease and delight than you ever dreamed possible. Soon you'll be improvising on your own, inventing your own recipes. Creativity's such a blast.

Imagine making delicious Brownies, chocolate sauce, chocolate mousse, frosting, or chocolate-drizzled cheesecake – all with *no sugar or fat*. Or the best fudge ice cream you've ever tasted: 70 calories per 1/2 cup serving, 0 g fat, 0 mg cholesterol, 8 carbs, & 0 g sugar. Imagine too: *pasta with 1/30th the carbs (Fettucini Alfredo!);* chocolate cookies[2], Anytime Brownies and Blondies[3] TM with No sugar, No fat, & *19 g. protein* per serving...& Pancakes[4] with everything bad replaced. Or Fat Free Mozzarella & Ricotta; sugar-free maple syrup; tuna or chicken salad with your homemade Mayonnaise Replacement that looks & *tastes* like mayonnaise. This book contains the recipes, plus a list of New Food Products needed to make them. And trust that everything here is delicious; impossible to tell from the "real" full-of-fat-and-sugar-metabolic-poison old thing. I'm a sugar fiend foodie as bad as anyone. My husband Bob, who's seen too much Sad in his cardiology practice, is more disciplined.

"I try!" he just said from a few feet away. He's writing furiously, and wants to speak to you next.

So quickly, and chocolate aside, trust too that this diet is common sense. No "eat-all-you-want-&-still-lose-weight" false promises. Starting on page 134 I'll show you current Diets, underlining, on

2   Recipe, p. 167, including ORAC stats bottom page.
      Read too p. 166 for ingredients NOT to use.

3   Low cal too. (All recipes are in the Index.)

4   Recipe, p. 89. It's funny.

each left page, <u>their unhealthy ingredients</u>…or the fact that, even if they start well, their entrées are so tiny that they leave you ravenous for their tiny NOT-for-dieters desserts. On the right pages I'll show you how to use new, healthy products to replace and *add*; *make bigger portions because you can*! Now to backtrack …

The problem with Low Carb/High Fat Diets: all that saturated fat. The problem with High Carb/ Low Fat Diets: all those carbs metabolize into sugar anyway, & too much sugar converts into fat. Plus they don't tell you that some carbs are fine (veggies, most fruits), and some bad & badder (white flour, corn, potato, rice, pasta, sugar, brown sugar, & couscous – just another flour with its husk removed). Some fats are healthy (mono- & poly-unsaturates), and some are nasty -- saturated and, worse, trans fats.

Beware too of food products now claiming **No Trans Fat!** [5] -- they're still sneaking in trans fats and saturated fats. Or claiming no saturated fat but their stuff is full of hidden sugars; or they claim no sugar but they're high in fat. Round and round. All carbs metabolize into sugar (some take an hour longer, true). <u>Metabolism's bottom line: EVERYTHING</u>[6] <u>breaks down to *just* one of three things: protein, fat, or sugar.</u> Lose the fat *or* the sugar -- even the "innocent natural sweeteners[7]" -- same game. Have you noticed that "diet products/programs" proclaim either No Fat or No Sugar; *never both?* Check them again. You'll see.

Even earnest diabetic sites claim no-sugar recipes -- but, unaware, they substitute brown sugar and crammed-with-sugar dates, bananas, molasses, honey, & evaporated fat free milk (one 12-oz can

---

5   See pages 51-52 & 160.

6   **"Good carbs, bad carbs?"** Right, up to a point, since some metabolize too fast. But they all still metabolize (maybe an hour later) to sugar, which, if there's too much, converts to fat.

7   Corn and agave have the highest sugar content of vegetables. Dates are the most sugar-crammed fruit. Next come raisins and *ripened* bananas. (The ripening process involves starch breaking down into sugar).

has 45 g carbs which quickly break down to 11 tsp sugar[8] – that's a candy bar!) That's how commercial diets keep the sugar hidden. Which is easy – people think sugar's just those little white granules in the sugar bowl.

The "big name" diets are unconscionable, Bob says. You know them. They advertise everywhere. Hire celebrities to tell you how great they are, and they all cost money to join. If something sounds too good to be true...

And those diets just count calories. Hey, you can lose weight on Snickers if you keep them down to 1,200 calories a day. Years ago in college I had an overweight friend who during the summer lost 40 pounds on chocolate éclairs. Just two a day, and beer. She returned in the fall looking wasted. Emaciated and sick, just awful. Wound up at the school infirmary.

Unfortunately -- & I've researched this online, in print, everywhere – the big business diets still have you eating the Worst Three: 1) sugar/brown sugar, 2) egg yolks/animal fats, 3) white flour.

If you're already protesting – right, right -- they tell you to use Splenda here and egg whites there, and be sure to spray with Pam before you broil your... "lean" pork & sirloin[9]. *Nooo! Animal fat is animal fat! One egg yolk has 300 mg. of cholesterol!* It's painful reading their recipes.

But not painful, if you know how I replace with New Products... creating eats just as delicious & vastly more healthy. Here's an example for simple Apple Crisp: on the left I've underlined the villains, and on the right, shown what I've replaced them with. In the Index you'll find the full recipe listed.

---

8   Every 4 g carbs = 1 teaspoon of sugar. (Take # of carbs, divide by 4.)

9   Even if you can't see the fat it's still there, in and around the cells of red meat.

- 4 sliced tart apples
- 3/4 cup brown sugar
- 1 cup all purpose flour
- 1/2 cup butter, softened
- 3/4 ground cinnamon
- 3/4 ground nutmeg
Per Serving, 512 calories

- 4 medium sliced tart apples
- 1 jar Sugar-Free Strawberry Preserves
- 1/4 cup Splenda
- 2 Minute Maid 'Just 10' Fruit punch [10 calories]
- 1/4 cup Whole Wheat Pastry Flour
- 1/4 cup Whole Grain Soy Flour
- *1 1/2 cups *milled* flaxseed, which also lowers your LDI (flaxseed replaces butter, oils in baking @ ratio of 3 to 1; also lowers your LDL, L for the Lousy one.)
Per serving, 113 calories

See? Create anything just as delicious with zero guilt? Top it with Sugar-Free Fat-Free Ice Cream at 35 calories per 1/4 cup. Add Fudge Syrup on top of the ice cream on top of the apple crisp, & it's a grand splurge of 160 calories with nothing bad in it. (But the crisp alone is terrific.)

And if the recipe had called for egg yolks? Use egg substitutes. One is Ener-G Egg Replacer -- good if the recipe calls for two or more yolks. If only 1 yolk is required (meaning it's only needed for binding), use 1 tablespoon baking powder, 1 tablespoon canola oil, and 1 tablespoon warm water.

Soy[10] can also substitute for egg yolks (1 yolk = 1 tablespoon soy flour + 1 tablespoon water). It has a huge amount of protein, can thicken gravies, and helps replace white flour which metabolizes almost as fast as sugar.

Something else: there's a new "soy margarine" product on the market. Forget it. It's nice about the soy, but the saturated fat they use? (Without saturated fat it wouldn't be solid at room

---

10 Soy contains complete protein with all the amino acids essential to human nutrition. It can lower your LDL cholesterol, & reduce the risk of heart disease and cancer. 1/4 cup soy flour = 25 g protein.

temperature.) Anyway, here's what they say about their wonderful saturated fat: "…while fats from coconut oil and palm kernel oil are [bad for you], we use the oil from the *fruit of the palm tree…*" Whoa! As Bob just told me, oil from the palm tree is the "least bad of the most terrible." Avoid that one.

With so much harmful misinformation on the web & in print, I urge you to make friends with the <u>Harvard School of Public Health Nutrition Source.</u> Google it. Study it. There's no better source, and its "Ask the Expert" is none other than Dr. Walter Willett, Harvard's Professor of Epidemiology and Nutrition, and an author of Harvard's famous paper – published in May of 1994! -- trying to warn the country about trans fats.

No…one…listened. Not the government, not the FDA, and certainly not restaurants and food manufacturers. Bob will tell you more about that in the next chapter.

A reminder: people's medical histories vary, and no diet book is the same as advice from your own physician. Check with him or her before embarking on any new weight loss and exercise program.

So here we go. In the pages ahead you'll find wonderful new diet recipes, chocolate's daily emotional/physical support, and the most honest, get-happily-thin-*and*-healthy information anywhere. I hope you make it a permanent part of your life.

Now Bob wants to talk to you.

The word "atherosclerosis[11]" comes from the Greek, athero, for porridge. So if you're ever in Greece & want porridge, say "Athero, hold the sclerosis!

CHAPTER TWO
America: the Shock

As a young physician, I took it for granted that America was the healthiest country on earth. Because it was. Widespread famine, contagion, and rampant epidemics were tragedies that happened elsewhere. We used to travel a lot, and see *preventable* disease that I'd only read about in textbooks. It was heartbreaking.

Like the time Joyce and I were in India. Walking the streets of New Delhi was like opening the pages of a med school textbook, seeing conditions I'd only read about but never dreamed I'd see. People with elephantiasis, children with kwashiorkor and trachoma. All so treatable! I trained at Bellevue, by the way, and thought I'd seen everything. I was still shocked.

Now America's the shock.

Bad enough to know the latest, awful statistics, but on every street: fat bellies, their owners blissfully unaware of their deterioration to come. With a glance I can spot the pre-diabetics and those who are already diabetic. That's a miserable feeling. I love this country. I can't believe this is happening.

11   See p. 140

One third of Americans will soon be diabetic, and another third pre-diabetic (glucose intolerant), with both groups facing futures marked by blindness, kidney failure, heart attacks, strokes, and amputations (gangrene from diabetes).

Is this any way to start a diet book? People just want to be beautiful, feel better -- not worse and scared as I've probably just scared you.

But maybe a little fear is good. It wakes us up. Shakes us from our complacency. Those diets "just to lose weight" may have been fine until the '90s. But in the last 15 years, the food we've been loving, becoming psychologically "addicted" to, has been monkeyed with, Frankensteinized (not too strong a word). It's done us real harm too.

To explain that I'll backtrack. Tell you things you may not have known...

• • •

Undo the harm...

[May 1994, research findings of the Harvard School of Public Health, appearing in the American Journal of Public Health]:

"...egregiously deceptive labels such as 'cholesterol-free' and 'cooked in vegetable oil.' ...the number of deaths attributable to such fats is likely to be substantial. Warning labels are more justifiable than those on cigarettes. We favor strict limitation of partially hydrogenated fat. Federal regulations should require manufacturers to include trans fatty content in food labels and should aim to greatly reduce or eliminate the use of partially hydrogenated vegetable fats."

1994! I saw Harvard's article re-printed again and again throughout the medical literature. Many physicians tried to warn their patients, as I did. But Americans receiving poor or no advice continued happily gobbling cookies and cakes and processed and junk foods. Because they didn't know.

In 2004, ten years later, the American Diabetes Association reported that cancer, diabetes and heart disease combined accounted for an astonishing two out of every three deaths in the United States (about 1.5 million a year). The following year brought worse numbers: 3,000 Americans died *each day* of cardiovascular disease – an average of one death every 25 seconds.

In 2006, twelve years after Harvard sounded the alarm, the FDA finally decided that trans fat should be listed on food labels. Food manufacturers started hustling to get the stuff out (largely replacing it with saturated fats, which I'll go into later). Hotels and restaurants started claiming to serve healthier food, and New York City set about becoming the first city in the country to limit trans fats in restaurants. Surprise: that proposal met fierce resistance from restaurant owners. Trans fats, you see, are *cheaper* than good fats (poly- and mono-unsaturated). "I'm wondering if there are grounds for a lawsuit," an official of the New York State Restaurant Association told the New York Times on September 27, 2006.

Those twelve years also produced many diet books, some of them even written by physicians (!?), with most of them continuing to say it was *okay* to eat that trans fatty margerine or butter substitute or full-of-lard "diet" or "meal replacement" bar. Sure -- smear it on your steak and bacon and egg yolks! Call me when you need bypass surgery.

Information was either absent, wrong or downright harmful. Trans fats blocked and inflamed the arteries of *even thin people*. Their LDLs climbed, their HDLs fell. (LDL's the bad one: think L for Lousy, H for healthy.) Harm happened to children too, and a new term entered our culture: Metabolic Syndrome, medical shorthand for high blood pressure, high cholesterol & triglycerides, central obesity (fat on the belly, the most dangerous place), diabetes, and heart disease.

Walking the streets, I can spot every diabetic and pre-diabetic. Worse, I know the exact future course of their medical histories. It's awful, and getting worse. You see overweight people too, but you can't picture their insides -- or your own. If you could, maybe you too would start getting a certain recurrent image in your mind. Something like thousands, millions of getting-sicker people with their heads in the sand.

Another shock

Today, in mid-December of 2006, is not a terrific day, because I just had another shock.

Diets: So many names, elaborate claims. I never paid attention to them but assumed that if an ad *said* something was a diet…it sort of was. Joyce hooted laughter and told me to read some of the diet books; go online to see their web sites too.

I could not believe my eyes.

First, I opened a "big name" diet book. The page I found at random had a recipe for chocolate cake: 3/4 cup of sugar, 3 egg yolks, 1 cup of flour, 3 tablespoons of butter, 1 1/2 ounces of chocolate, and 2 tablespoons of vegetable shortening. *What? Was this possible?* I re-checked the book title to make sure I hadn't picked up the wrong book. Nope, the title really said DIET. But the page I'd found was a recipe to *gain* weight, worsen diabetes, block your arteries!

And the serving size was miniscule. Even if you only ate that tiny piece, you'd just consumed 200 calories crammed with 4 grams of saturated fat (9 total fat) and 30 grams of carbs.

Right there's another trick, just quoting the "30 grams of carbs." Nowhere did the recipe or nutritional facts give the sugar content.

Plus, can we assume there were no trans fats? Maybe, but it didn't say -- and in any case, if the trans fats were taken out they were clearly replaced with saturated fat.

Next, I went online to sites of different but equally "big" diets. Yow. Here's a typical "lose weight" recipe for brownies: 3/4 cup flour, 1/2 cup of chocolate chips, 6 tablespoons of butter, 1/2 cup of applesauce, and 2 eggs (including yolks).

100 calories! exclaimed the sales talk, but again the serving was tiny – and who eats just one? Also again, nowhere did it give the saturated fat, trans fat, or sugar content.

I spent hours going through all the diet books and web sites, and then sat back, incredulous. This…is unconscionable! Such recipes in so-called "diet" books and "diet programs?" Is there any diet at all that has worked in the long run? Obesity & diabetes are skyrocketing faster. There's your answer.

• • •

"Speed Up Your Metabolism?"

I googled the above & got more than a million hits. Mostly people trying to sell you something, most not even knowing what the word metabolism means. *It doesn't mean burning calories faster.* That's the misconception.

Your thyroid rules metabolism, and sets the rate at which your muscles – repeat, muscles – turn sugar and fat into energy (burn calories). No pill or magic drink is going to speed up that Basal Metabolic Rate (BMR)…but you *can* use up more calories by exercise.

Muscles are our machinery. Picture two guys working out, hefting the same-weight barbells at the same intense rate. One is muscular, devoted to exercise & working out; the other is skinny & just starting (or his muscles are skinny under lots of fat). They're doing the exact same thing -- but who's burning more calories? The muscular one. Our bodies are like cars: the bigger, heavier ones use more fuel. Remember <u>metabolism's bottom line: EVERYTHING breaks down to just one of three things: protein, fat, or sugar</u>. Even in wacky theory, what's the difference if that fat or sugar reaches your liver a half hour earlier? It will still turn to fat & high blood sugar *if there's too much of it.*

"Speed Up Your Metabolism" just means another frustrating gimmick. Don't waste your money.

• • •

Our diet for life

Now I'll go back, way back, to the early 1980s. Our children were small, my wife Joyce was working on her first novel, and I, a cardiologist concerned about the already-spiking rate of coronary disease, would come home each night with the latest scoop on diet and nutrition from The New England Journal of Medicine, The American Journal of Cardiology, and everything else in the medical literature. "Oops," I'd say, "Ease off on red meat," and, "Better start cooking with olive oil." So Joyce made it practically a game to understand, then duplicate recipes we found in any restaurant into meals just as delicious, artistic, low-cal and heart smart. That's how she's been cooking ever since -- though just 2 or 3 times a week -- since, like everyone else, she has little time to cook. And when she does get out the skillets she makes enough for a regiment, then freezes it for...whenever.

That's how it started, this diet-for-life of ours. Don't worry: it recognizes that the occasional "cheat" or even binge is normal. Did I mention that we're really closet junk food junkies? Who isn't? There was even a time when our idea of fun was staging raids on the CVS candy aisle – Joyce will laugh and tell you she's a worse binger; I'd feebly try to pull her away from the chocolate and wind up flinging off Hershey wrappers too. But the next day it would be, "Okay, penance! Back to broccoli and exercise!"

That's how it's been for 98% of each year. We look and feel decades younger, with energy and blood chemistries to match. We almost feel like a science experiment ☺.

As a clinical cardiologist of thirty years' experience I can't emphasize it enough: this is a both a diet to lose weight, and a health program for a lifetime. The recipes are easy, crammed with nutrients, and if you cheat just go back to it the next day. I urge you to share it with and teach it to your loved ones.

• • •

Amazing Facts...

1. Your blood sugar drops with just a 1-pound weight loss. In fact, with just the first *ounces* off, you've made yourself immediately healthier. (Overweight is also a huge risk factor for breast and ovarian cancer in women, prostate cancer in men, and colon cancer in both men and women.)

2. Your heart, which is the size of your closed fist, is a small, overworked muscle, pumping 24/7. *And for every extra pound of fat you carry, your body has to grow seven new miles of blood vessels--* primarily capillaries but also small arteries (arterioles) and small veins (venules) -- and your heart has to work that much harder. Put on two pounds and that's fourteen new miles of blood vessels; fifty extra pounds requires 350 miles of new blood vessels. On and on, do the math.

But good news: the opposite is true. For every pound of fat you lose, your body sheds seven miles of blood vessels. They just re-absorb, break down, and get excreted. Lose two pounds and that's fourteen miles of blood vessels gone, lightening your heart's load.

I've told you these two things so you'll know that even a little is a lot. Repeat that out loud to yourself: *even a little is a lot.* Let it be your mantra.

Because dieting is a slooow process, like watching the grass grow. Try to accept that, and the next time you catch yourself groaning, "Oh it's almost a week and I've only lost two pounds" – understand that that's *good*. You've already brought valuable change to your body; taken a literal load off your heart. Try this too for reinforcement: take a can off the shelf that weighs one or two pounds, and heft it. Or, in the supermarket, keeping your elbow straight, lift some wrapped meat weighing two pounds. It's *heavy*. And you'll think, Wow, I lost *this* much?

Now, here's Joyce. We'll be taking turns; I have more to tell you. But first hear about her recipes and list of fantastic New-Age food products, and the jammed, crammed freezer, and tonight's chicken fettuccini and chocolate pudding with walnuts and sliced strawberries.

This is all making me hungry…

CHAPTER THREE
How This Evolved

Hello again, Diet Marine,

That just popped into my head. I don't think it's corny. There are different ways of being brave.

I have so been there: up and down with the weight, the love handles, avoiding the scale and the jeans I couldn't pull past my knees. But I was also lucky: Bob is a cardiologist, one of those M.D.s who first specialize in Internal Medicine, and then subspecialize in diseases of the heart and blood vessels. He's also a thin cardiologist who wanted to stay that way, so decades ago, with his coaching, I started cooking in a different way.

For a second I want to go back to something I just said: that Bob, for thirty years, has practiced *both* Internal Medicine and Cardiology. This is an important distinction. It means that he was treating diseases of the whole body, including overweight, high blood pressure, cholesterol, coronary disease, and diabetes all along. He saw the diabetes epidemic happening years before it became an obsessive topic. He tried to caution every patient, succeeded with some, came home shaking his head about others.

Just ran downstairs to get a few terms re-dictated; Bob's making heart-smart soy & flaxseed pancakes with delicious sugar-free maple syrup. Now I'm back, but wait – did you know that the "good" polyunsaturated fats in flaxseed[12] are high in alpha-linolenic acid (an omega-3 fatty acid)? It prevents serious heart problems.

I'm getting ahead of myself, but wanted to give you an idea of the New Healthy Food Products and how I'll teach you to use them. I've made a list of them for you on p. 57.

But okay, what's the crucial difference between an Internist/ Cardiologist and someone who *just* practices cardiology?

In a word, the person who practices just cardiology gets the patient when s/he's already sick. The correct term is Invasive Cardiologist: someone who confines his or her practice to in-hospital testing such as stress thallium tests, angiograms (imaging arteries' interiors), angioplasty (a balloon pushed through arteries to try to clear them), and IVUS, or intravascular ultrasound. That cardiologist treats patients who already have coronary disease, and will see them only briefly.

Whereas the Internist/Cardiologist knows his patients for years, decades, and tries to keep them well so they won't *need* the Invasive Cardiologist.

Some listen, many don't. For a while I was among those who didn't. I'd only gain 10 or 12 pounds at a time, but I'd go around moaning about it, concerned with what just the *outside* of me looked like, and Bob taught me how to turn it around. But something else began to change. I started peeking at those medical journals, asking what this meant, and that meant, and starting to get impressed. Scared, even. The photos did it: pictures in The New England Journal of Medicine and The American Journal of Cardiology of arteries so

---

12 Get *Milled* flaxseed, online if not locally. Un-milled isn't absorbed by the body. HodgsonMill.com & BobsRedMill.com are good sources.

gunked they looked like the Roto-Rooter ad; pictures of human hearts (after autopsy) *encased* in fat! Yes, it was gross, revolting. As that movie tag-line goes, Be afraid, be very afraid...

I'll repeat what Bob said. A little fear is good. It wakes us up.

I was never hooked on cheeseburgers, etc., but the seeming impossible battle with my sweet tooth continued. By the late eighties, though, I knew well that cheating meant more than just getting pudgy. There were still times in the supermarket when I could not...push the cart...past...the gorgeous array behind the see-through bakery doors, but when Bob got home I'd be like some Peanuts cartoon wailing, *"Argh-h, I just committed suicide by cookie!"*

So I re-lost the weight. And got more disciplined -- such an old-fashioned word! Who wants that when we can have instant gratification!

But a strange, unconscious thing happened. Each time I lost weight, and stayed with the program longer...I *stopped thinking* about sweets. Really. It just happened. The first week or more was hard, but the longer I went without my beloved cookies and candy, the more they became just an abstraction, something I forgot to think about. Like an itch I toughed out not scratching...and it went away. That was the biggest revelation. The big secret of how successful weight losers have done it. The longer you tough it out the easier it gets; the whole *obsession* lets go. You've changed your psychology. Shut down your cravings. Learned you don't have to be constantly chomping on something. Established a whole new relationship with food.

That is how you'll lose weight. And have, at least 98% of the time for the rest of your life, a healthier way of eating.

Don't clutch, or imagine something hugely ambitious, do-or-die -- and why, pray tell, has losing weight been made into such an over-complicated emotional thing? Sure, dieting is hard, like any discipline. And as Bob said a few pages ago, some diets we now know were unsafe, with built-in "failure" trip-ups and resulting anxiety. This cannot have been their authors' intention. But the most recent discoveries in Nutrition and Cardiology have changed everything, with trans fat damage and the obesity epidemic telling us how badly diets of the last decade have backfired. The fact that you hold this book in your hands shows how unhelpful they were.

Take a deep breath, and close your eyes for a moment. Hang in there with me.

Besides the new-age healthy foods, I'm going to teach you low-cal, heart-smart *MLA (Make Lots Ahead) recipes I've been using all along. Each is delicious, filling, and Extreme Anti-oxidant. Nutrients crammed into every gram. And since I see no need for those silly "phase 1," "phase 2" detox-starve-yourself gimmicks (how they misuse the word "detox"), these recipes also, from day one, use all three food groups: carbs, fat, and protein; chicken, fish, olive oil, nuts, fresh fruits, and vegetables.

And you can still have fun or binge occasionally. Once a week steak or other red meat is okay. If we were perfect, non-craving robots, it would be better *not* to, but do your best. Just know, as I did in my suicide-by-cookie days, that there are no free rides, and do "penance" the next day. Back to broccoli and exercise. And try not to let stress, which everyone has in their life, pull you down.

What about snacks? Those late-afternoon, late-evening "droopies" are hard. Right, agreed. Fruit and nuts are fine, but go easy on the fruits, they're full of sugar. Walnuts, by the way, are super good for you, containing the same omega-3 acids that flaxseed and salmon & tuna do. One handful of walnuts and almonds is filling and terrific. Watch out, though: they taste too good; there's the danger of losing control.

Here's another danger. *Few dieters want to accept the trade-off.* Their biggest complaint about the cookie or whatever is, "This doesn't taste like the real thing." Well of course it doesn't! It's the fat & sugar that made it taste so good. So take your choice: Continue eating what's more delicious, keel over 30 years earlier – getting sick and sicker in the meantime – or lose the pounds and binge only rarely.

Think of the Tom Hanks character in "CASTAWAY."

I was about to stop but something else just got me mad. On the web, have you seen those "Lose 9 pounds in 11 days" ads? Sigh-h. How *do* people get away with such harmful nonsense? Here's why such a claim is not even physically possible.

A typical person needs 2,000 calories a day. Ok, let's starve them. Give them only water, and 0 calories a day. Got a calculator? Eleven days of not eating equals 2,000 times 11 or a 22,000 deficit. And each pound equals 3,500 calories -- so 22,000 divided by 3,500 = 6.28 pounds. Six and one-quarter pounds, that's it, the maximum possible real weight loss by starving for eleven days. Even if someone starting at, say, 300 pounds loses as much as 8 or 9 pounds in those first eleven days (most of it water), in *subsequent* 11-day periods, 6 1/4 pounds will become the maximum weight lost...by not eating at all. Total starvation. So much for harmful misinformation on the 'net.

Losing weight correctly isn't some crash program, but a long process. Just remember Bob's *"for every extra pound of fat you carry, your body has to grow seven new miles of blood vessels."* And the opposite: For every pound of fat you lose, your body *sheds* seven miles of blood vessels. One pound – and your heart, your whole body is instantly healthier!

Realizing this will help you persevere.

A minute ago Bob gave me a New Age Pancake (no eggs, no bad flour, no sugar or its invisible substitutes) rolled up with chopped walnuts and Philadelphia Fat Free Cream Cheese (15 calories per tablespoon). I'm going to run down for maple syrup (Log Cabin Sugar Free, 35 calories per *1/4 cup*). He'll take the wheel now to give you more information, tips, and fascinating insights.

CHAPTER FOUR
More Information and Tips

Genetically, we human beings probably weren't intended to eat anything more than nuts and berries. That's pretty much what our distant ancestors subsisted on, to be replaced in later centuries by food they had to labor to grow, and then cook (after chopping the firewood), and then try to preserve through the winter. So most people were thin. Even into the 1960s and 70s most people were thin, and obesity was a rarity.

Now we're surrounded by all this delicious *stuff*. No labor. Yummies in a bag you can just stick your hand into. If it had existed 100 or 1,000 years ago, they would have been fat too. We're only human -- what to do?

We fear terrorists, but we're killing ourselves at the rate of 3,000 a *day* with cancer, diabetes and heart disease. As Joyce just said, Be afraid… It's not a bad way to start; that concern's more statistically realistic.

Many have told me they've tried every diet, and *it* didn't work for *them*. Flawed diets, yes, it's understandable. But many have also told me they're addicted to food, or that they've inherited the "fat gene." The media like to use these terms, because it makes us happy, gives us an excuse, and we'll continue watching their stations and buying their magazines.

But no. Even the most compulsive over-eating doesn't, medically speaking, constitute true physical addiction, with withdrawal including shakes, sweats, and hallucinations (have you ever actually seen someone going through withdrawal?). And for those with the "fat gene," I mean no offense, but would be curious to see photos of their grandparents.

Which brings us back to the question, What to do?

There's an old saying you may have heard: Sow an action and you reap a habit. Sow a habit and you reap a destiny.

Thus the place to begin is, sow an action. Just one. Drive past the McDonald's or Dunkin' Donuts or Pizza Hut without stopping. Or resist the temptation of those cookies at your neighbor's or in the supermarket. That's it. You've sown your first action. It will give you confidence in yourself. Do it again, and the feeling will grow.

Here's a tip: Look at that cake or junk food and imagine how you'll feel *after* you eat it, not while.

• • •

Learn how to shut off the cravings.

When you start eating less, your body will automatically switch gears. Give it just under a week: it will register that your glycogen is depleted, and start breaking down your stored fat for energy. Genetically, this is how our bodies adapted to times of famine. And how do you activate this response? Just tough it out for a few days. Then your body -- your liver, actually, which is the Houston Control of your metabolism -- will switch from your old up-down, glucose-insulin pattern to one where you're steadily breaking down fat. You'll feel this as your cravings shutting down. It gets easier as you learn to substitute foods which will last you longer for those which were causing your insulin highs, lows, and crashes. This is how you'll redesign your own glucose pattern. It's an empowering feeling.

Fructose,[13] *the New Danger:*

Just another member of the sugar family, but fructose is not safe, especially in quantity. It's the biggest bait-and-switch gimmick in years. A derivative of honey, berries, tree fruits, agave (90% fructose), & sweet potatoes, fructose has been commercialized into a refined sugar which -- true, absorbs more slowly, but also damages the body far more. Fructose & HFCS (high-fructose corn syrup) have been added to processed foods, beverages and, more ominously, so-called "diet yummies," telling people they can "cheat & eat" as much as they like. Irony: fructose, with its longer shelf life & the fact that it's cheaper, *has become the trans fat of the sugar family.* (For more, google "dangers of fructose.")

What about Stevia? Another controversy. The FDA has refused to approve stevia because of its possible cancer-causing effects. Pro-stevians argue that it's been used by South American natives for centuries, without mentioning how long those people *lived* (not counting battles, snakes bites, animal attacks, & infectious disease). Also, were any long-term studies & control group studies done on them? Cancer can take years to develop, as with smoking. Meanwhile stevia's being as aggressively marketed as fructose.

• • •

13   In addition to causing the old white sugar health problems, fructose can cause blood clots, liver & heart muscle damage, insulin resistance/diabetes, accelerate aging, interfere with the immune system, and lead to osteoporosis. It also raises your LDL by disrupting liver metabolism. Fructose and Trans Fats are both worse than what they were supposed to replace in their ability to cause disease.

What are Sugar Alcohols?

There are five main sweeteners in commercial use today: saccharin, aspartame, sucralose, acesulfame, and sugar alcohols. "Sugar alcohols," a consumer-friendly name, are derived but changed from sugar molecules, and include names like sorbitol, mannitol, xylitol, lactitol, maltitol, and others. They still have calories of the sugar type (though fewer: 2-3 calories per gram as opposed to 4 calories per gram of standard sugar), but they still affect your blood sugar and are no free ride, especially for diabetics. Their benefit is that they metabolize more slowly than regular sugar, so they last you longer, hold off those need-sweets-again-crashes.

Products containing sugar alcohols are marketed as "no sugar added" -- but beware. They often cause bloating and diarrhea. There is also the misconception that all sugar alcohol-containing products are "sugar free." These products may still contain significant amounts of carbohydrates, which break down to sugar anyway. Check the labels.

Sugar alcohols vs. Artificial Sweeteners

Sugar alcohols and artificial sweeteners, such as saccharin (Sweet & Low) and aspartame (Equal, NutraSweet, and NatraTaste) are not the same. Artificial sweeteners contain no calories or carbohydrates at all.

Saccharin got a bad rap a few years ago – it produced bladder cancer in rats exposed to prodigious amounts – but those tests didn't hold up in humans (no one would eat a truckload of saccharin). Still, it seems to have a slightly metallic aftertaste.

Instead we like aspartame, and love Splenda - which is only 1% sucralose which is itself FDA-approved. Aspartame is in Diet Coke, practically everything else, and we've experienced no side effects from either aspartame or Splenda. Both have decades-long track records and many studies in humans: no red flags, as physicians say.

Now you're wondering, if Splenda and aspartame are so great, why do manufacturers still use sugar alcohols? Because only sugar, in one form or another, makes the cookie stiff, the gum or candy bulky. Splenda and aspartame are terrific in your coffee or no-fat yogurt or to bake with (Splenda), but they can't make the muffin bind, the cookie stiff. That's why, since trans fats have been banished, you'll find sugar alcohols in more and more products. And sugar alcohols are still technically carbohydrates, remember. Check the labels.

They're still a boon, though, these artificial sweeteners -- and, in moderation, sugar alcohols. The average American consumes *142 pounds of sugar per year*, up from 100 pounds 30 years ago. There is a staggering amount of sugar in certain products: soft drinks, pies, cookies, cakes, candy, ice cream, etc. A typical can of a non-diet soft drink contains 40 - 50 grams of sugar, the equivalent of 12 teaspoons. Ten soft drinks per day, not unusual for a teenager, equals a pound of sugar; just five cans equal a half-pound of sugar.

Is there any doubt about the contribution of sugar (including carbs broken down to sugar) to the epidemic of obesity and diabetes in kids? The health wreckage in adults?

· · ·

Listen through My Stethoscope

In the normal heart, what you hear with each heartbeat is a "lub dub." Two sounds per beat, with pure silence between them. That silence is called systole.

Now listen to the heart of this 55-year-old man, overweight for years but jovial, unconcerned. Place the stethoscope over his heart, and in a millisecond you'll hear…the ping! of diagnosis, the feeling a physician gets when there's a sudden physical finding s/he knows will change a patient's life.

It is the characteristic loud rasping of an aortic systolic murmur. An ugly sound, just dreadful. That systole should be clean! Silent! Not sound like dragging a butter knife over a cheese grater. But there it is, again. And again. A lifetime of too much food high in sugar and saturated fat. The finding hasn't quite sunk in for this patient, but he's somber. Says that doctors "begged him for years" to lose weight. And he tried, but it was haaard, and fun was better. Over time, cholesterol layered on his aortic valve, followed by calcium deposition. The delicate valve leaflets became "glued" together, narrowing the space through which oxygenated blood is pumped by his heart to other body organs. If this stenosis (narrowing) isn't caught and diagnosed, it will worsen silently, causing crippling or lethal strokes. This patient will have to undergo aortic valve replacement, a major operation with all its pain and risks, and a lifetime of medications and close medical supervision.

That sound that came through the stethoscope? I call it the sound of the Fed Too Wells. *And today we have all the diseases of the Fed-Too-Wells down through history.*

• • •

Only the Rich Used to be Fed-Too-Wells

Not everyone in history was thin. There was always that 1% of every culture, the rich, who got the diseases now rampant in America and the West (Europe too). In the 18th & 19th centuries, the girth of a man's paunch was a measure of his wealth. And only the wealthy got gout, a painful arthritic condition caused by fatty meats. Known for centuries as "the disease of kings," gout has been studied intently by physicians since the days of Hippocrates. Henry VIII was only 56 when he died. Hans Holbein painted the portrait opposite of him in 1537, when Henry was 46. What a picture of arrogance and power -- but he looks fat and old too. He ate hugely: oily red meats, few vegetables (which were considered food for the poor), and sweets made with honey and fat drippings (bread puddings were baked under the roasting, dripping meats). For sure he had high blood pressure and clogged arteries. Between his mid- and late forties he went from a 37-inch waist & 45-inch chest to a staggering 54-inch waist and 57-inch chest. He suffered "grieviously" from leg ulcers and bulging varicose veins, and died of breathing problems and an infected leg.

Here is the medical sequence: central obesity (fat belly) causes pressure on the abdominal veins, which transmits down the legs, causing bulging varicose veins. Clots form in the leg veins (phlebitis), break loose, travel to the lungs, and cause a pulmonary embolism. This chain of events is predictable, and still frequent.

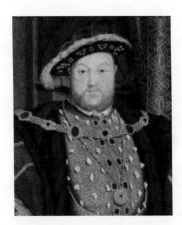

Beware the LDL train

LDL is the dirty Litter train. It leaves Metabolism Central – the liver -- and begins its circuit dumping sticky, revolting cholesterol in every artery. Finished, it returns through the veins to the liver where it picks up another load. Back and forth, dumping and clogging…as long as the liver's owner keeps supplying it with fat and cholesterol.

HDL, the Healthy train, is meanwhile traveling the same artery tracks, trying to clean up. An exhausting job, with all that burger and cupcake mush squeezing into the intestines -- worse, pushing HDL *down* and LDL *up*. Outnumbered! But HDL struggles on, trying to clean tracks disappearing into the muck.

Then, one day, something happens. LDL returns to the liver and finds -- what's this? *Less fat?* Glycogen depleting, starting to break down stored fat for energy? Because it's owner's *on a diet?* Nooo!

Yes, says HDL, suddenly stronger. OUTTA MY WAY. Fast, the HDL train makes enough clean-up trips to fill the town dump…

• • •

Younger Plaque is More Dangerous

Here's a surprise: older plaque lining your arteries, blocking them even up to 90%, is *less* likely to cause an acute heart attack than new plaque which may block the artery only 20 or 30%. This is because old plaque has grown a tough, fibrous cap, or membrane. You lucked out there. But newer plaque, almost as soon as it's laid down, develops a delicate membrane which cracks easily as inflammation damages it and high blood pressure pounds it. Then the body's natural tendency to form a clot (like a scab) over damaged tissue can cause sudden, complete blockage of the artery. That part of the heart muscle is starved for oxygenated blood, and dies. Yes, a heart attack.

So. Even if you lucked out with the older plaque, there's damage done *last week* to arteries, and disaster could still strike unless you start dieting and exercising *today*. I truly don't mean to scare you, but you should know that problems are even more likely now, since the old plaque has already narrowed arteries and done invisible damage.

How do you keep that new plaque from forming at all? Sorry: it's only by diet and exercise. Some medications are wonderful, but very recent studies show that nothing's as good as exercise and losing weight to get that new, more dangerous plaque to re-absorb; i.e, get picked up by your HDL and taken to the liver, where it's broken down and excreted.

Gone! Thank you HDL. I'll start taking better care of you.

Statin Drugs

I've heard it a thousand times: *Gimme the pill, doc. Woo-hoo, no more need for lifestyle change!*

Statin drugs are, indeed, excellent. Even without dieting they'll lower your LDL and slightly raise your HDL, so that's good, right?

Yes BUT. Statins work on your cholesterol, but if you're overweight and sedentary, you're still prone to diabetes and high blood pressure -- and high blood pressure, remember, pounds the inner lining of your arteries, causing inflammation and cracks in the plaque membrane, which causes scabby clots and artery blockage, which then starve the heart muscle of oxygenated blood and kill that part of the heart muscle. Yes again, a heart attack.

Beware of considering any drug as a cure-all.

Obesity + sedentary = bad, bad, bad. You still must lose the weight and exercise. And in the process, hey -- you'll get more beautiful. Health *and* beauty! It's a win/win! You just have to do it...

• • •

Belly Bands

The current hot thing is the adjustable gastric lap band, which requires a laparoscopic insertion of the device. Laparoscopy involves making an incision in the abdominal wall, then, under local anesthesia and sedation, passing a tube through which the band is applied to the upper part of the stomach, limiting the amount of food which can be eaten at one time. The degree of tightness can be varied. Usually three incisions and three tubes are used: one to see through, one to manipulate instruments, one to pass the device and clean up inside the belly afterwards.

What are the risks? The same ones involved in any invasive procedure entering the abdominal cavity: reactions to the sedative or local anesthetic (or general anesthetic when used); intra-abdominal hemorrhage; infection (peritonitis, a very nasty kind of infection in the belly); laceration of intestine, stomach, gall bladder -- need I go on? Long term, what are the effects on nutrition, mood, overall health?

The band can also slip later, or erode the stomach wall. I don't like the statistic I've seen, that the MORTALITY RATE for the operation is "**as low as**" 1 in 2000. First, "as low as" means... higher. How *much* higher? 1 in 1,000? 1 in 500? They don't tell us. Second, that disclaimer doesn't count long term illness and death from possible post-op infections.

Aftercare is long and hard: band adjustments, nutrition and behavioral advice, frequent meetings with a counselor, support groups, telephone access to a support buddy. It's a full time job.

Despite all this, there's only about a 50% success rate. Five years later, only about half of the intended weight loss has been achieved. I wonder if the same result could be achieved just by the follow-up counseling program? Skip the surgery.

Hoodia

The good news about Hoodia: it does appear to suppress appetite.

The bad news: Hoodia, which comes from a plant (Hoodia gordonii) native to desert areas of South Africa, is very rare and protected by South Africa's conservation laws. The South African government has limited the export and farming of Hoodia to prevent over-exploitation -- and it is difficult to synthesize in the lab. The pharmaceutical giant, Pfizer, tried for several years to grow & market it, then gave up.

So there's no way Hoodia's being produced in the commercial quantity needed, and what's really being sold online is...I don't know. Some dried, powdered *substance* called hoodia, of which the FDA is wary, and may soon clamp down. These products are not regulated or inspected, and there are no published clinical trials to establish an optimal dose that is safe and effective. Many have even complained that the "supplements" they ordered didn't contain any Hoodia at all.

The only clinical study I'm aware of showed that Hoodia could present risks to organs, nervous and circulatory systems. Liver damage in particular was suspected.

The Latest 2 Things to Beware of:

Butter & margarine. Since the word about trans fat is out, I've noticed diets & diet magazines hustling back to butter, extolling "its old time natural goodness." Also margarines, many of which have put saturated fats back in because, without either trans fat or saturated fat, the margarine won't be *solid at room temperature.* Check the Nutrition Fact labels. If the fat figures are hidden (they do that) or don't add up-- and the margarine or whatever is solid at room temperature, that's not good.

(Certainly butter is delicious, mouth-watering just to think about. But you didn't see them telling you to use it back in the old trans fat days, did you?)

• • •

Amazing Epidemiolgy...What is it?

Epidemiology is the study of disease and disease history in large populations. It gives valuable clues to how our bodies work, and, in this case, how diet and exercise affect our health and longevity. Think of it as detective work. And consider these stories which took place after World War II:

1. After the war two men worked on a London double decker bus. One drove. The other, the conductor, climbed up and down the steps all day punching tickets of boarding passengers. Since the war ended each had packed the pounds back on, and were pretty evenly matched in terms of age, height, and weight. So...guess who rapidly developed heart disease and died? Yep, the driver. His conductor friend had come to the hospital in tears, telling their story. First one doctor and then several were intrigued, and a study widened to include thousands of "bus pairs" of

London Transit workers. Same thing. The first epidemiologic shocker on coronary disease, showing the incidence of heart attacks, angina, and sudden cardiac death to be much higher among drivers *who just sat* at their jobs, than among conductors who trudged up and down stairs each day.

2. The Norwegian diet, traditionally high in beef and dairy products, became one of near starvation during the brutal Nazi occupation. Ironically, and despite the horrendous stress of the time, the incidence of acute coronary disease plunged, only to rise again to its pre-war level after the war. Ruling out every variable, the only answer astonished scientists came up with was the absence of all that animal fat. Hence, the second early landmark discovery, now called the Oslo Wartime Coronary Disease Study.

3. The Japanese always had a low incidence of breast and colon cancer, and a high rate of stomach cancer. After the war many Japanese moved to the United States, and something strange happened: the disease profiles reversed. The next generation of Japanese-Americans became much more prone to breast and colon cancer, and less afflicted by stomach cancer – quickly resembling cancer rates and food habits of other Americans. Meanwhile data from Japan showed *no change there*, which clinched it for epidemiologists. The Japanese diet in Japan, though low in fat, is high in pickled food which leads to stomach cancer...while the high-fat American diet leads to colon and breast cancer.

Knowledge isn't just power, it's health. Some 60 years later, mountains of epidemiological evidence and statistically precise testing have reinforced our understanding, and it's clear: DIET is Number One in health and longevity. *You really are what you eat.* Keep the fats way down, and vary your diet.

Ahead is a list of bad and good foods; also more diet info and answers to commonly asked questions.

CHAPTER FIVE
Losin' It

Three Notes first

- It bears repeating: many diets have been "high-fat/low carb," or the reverse. That's nonsense. Because some carbs are fine (veggies, most fruits), and some bad (corn, potato, pasta, rice, sugar). Some fats are fine (mono- & poly-unsaturates), and some are nasty -- saturated and, worse, trans fats. ("Trans fats" are the same thing as hydrogenated fats. Hydrogenate refers to the Process; trans fats refers to the result of hydrogenation.) Also, *carbs break down to sugar anyway!* How misleading, for any diet to refer to carbs and sugar as if they're different. Pasta, rice or couscous – it all breaks down to sugar.

- And how wrongly the word "Natural" has been used. Beef fat is natural. So are heavy cream and sugar and pork fat and the majority of poisons.

- Some diets, while being honest about butter substitutes, said it was okay to eat egg *yolks*, and bacon, sausage, steak and different kinds of cheese. How we wish it were so! But it isn't. Animal fats are animal fats -- and *why* does a diet "allow you to cheat" when this guarantees you'll return to your old ways? Gain the weight right back instead of learning a new relationship to food? Why do some diets do this? Because they don't want you to get bored. And they want you to think you can "eat what you love and still lose weight!" And to tell your friends to buy their books, join their Buy-Only-Our-Food programs, order their full-of-lard "nutrition/diet/meal replacement"/ bars too. It's all big business.

• • •

Food idea rejected by McDonalds: Way Too Damn Happy Meal

1. First and obviously...**avoid Junk Food.** This is hard, at first. It's everywhere. Just when you're hungriest it's right there next to the cash register, or you're driving by it, or it's on the supermarket shelves and the TV ads. A barrage. I'll bet these junk food corporate types don't let their own children eat their stuff, but they make billions from us. And their shareholders are happy. Aren't we terrific for making their shareholders happy? Think in terms of the 5-day hump, which is what it takes for the "itch," the craving, to go away. So first, get through just one day of not stopping at Dunkin' Donuts, not buying that impulse sweet, not letting your kids whine you into that fast food place. *Just one day.* Then, do it again the next day, which makes...two whole days! And you know what? You'll be proud of yourself. You'll be thrilled with yourself in a way you haven't been for years. That feeling will carry you forward another day – wow, and another...and very soon, IT GETS EASIER. You can stick your nose up when you pass McDonald's and say "I'm strong, I don't *need* you! I've *kicked* you!" The bad-for-you goodies will start to become an abstraction, something you don't even see or think about anymore. At least not so obsessively. As with babies, it's a kind of weaning. (Have you seen the DVD, SUPERSIZE ME? You'll never want to look at a cheeseburger again.)

2. Avoid too: **Red Meats** (once a month or hardly ever); **hi-fat**

dairy (low fat or fat free OK); and **carbs** such as pasta, rice, potatoes, corn, bread, cereal, cakes, cookies, muffins, couscous, and sugar. Carbs raise blood sugar because all carbs metabolize (some more slowly, true) into sugar; excessive carbs are converted from sugar into fat. Also avoid egg **yolks**. Egg whites are invaluable, but *throw out the yolks*. Don't even give them to the dog -- every yolk contains 300 milligrams of bad cholesterol. Consider this: 300 mg. of cholesterol is the maximum "safe" daily amount for people with *no* cardiovascular risk factors. For people with one or two cardiovascular risk factors the maximum is 200 mg; and for people with three or more risk factors, the maximum amount is 100 mg. Again: one yolk = 300 milligrams, the maximum safe daily amount for, say, a 30-year-old skinny athlete. Research and medical science are constantly being updated, and doctors do change their party line. So this is the most up to date cardiology. Throw *out* the darn yolks.

3. What are the **cardiovascular risk factors**? Obesity, high blood pressure, high cholesterol & triglycerides, diabetes, prior history of cardiovascular disease, sedentary lifestyle, smoking, and family history of cardiovascular disease.

4. **Liquid egg whites**: Invaluable. Great for breakfast, lunch, and dinner recipes.

5. **Hydrogenated or partially hydrogenated:** What does it mean? To hydrogenate means to pass bubbling hydrogen through a tube into any unsaturated cooking oil. This turns the oily liquid into a solid at room temperature. Until 2006, it was sold to manufacturers of baked and processed foods, or colored yellow, sent to market where it would have a longer shelf life, and called a butter substitute – despite mounting evidence starting in the early 1990s that the substance was a killer. (Cf. Harvard's May 1994 study, p. 11.) If you were to hydrogenate olive oil, it would be just as bad for you. Since

2006 and the new legislation, you must still be careful. Manufacturers of margarine/spreads and baked and processed foods now gleefully report on their Nutrition Labels that there are **0 grams of hydrogenated**...*but have some switched back to using saturated fats (animal fats or palm oil)?* With too many it's the old shell game. Margarines and spreads MUST contain either saturated fat or hydrogenated/trans fats, or they'd be liquid at room temperature. Next time you shop, look at the "total fat" number, then look for the "saturated fat" numbers, and do the math. Missing saturated fat? Trans fat? And who eats just one teaspoon or one cookie? On everything you buy for the first time, check the labels. If the product contains either saturated or hydrogenated fats, skip it. Saturated fats are the second worst thing, and if you really want to clean out those arteries, stick to foods cooked with olive oil, canola oil, etc.

6. **Cheese.** One diet book we read said Well, you can eat mozzarella, parmesan, brie, and ricotta, but don't eat this one or this and this... Horsefeathers. Cheese is cheese, full of animal fat. However, you can use Fat Free Singles which come in cheddar, American, and white cheese flavor. (Kraft is one brand; they're a bit more expensive but worth it for your health, and an excellent product.) Joyce cooks, bakes, and makes sandwiches with these Fat Free Singles. And wait till you see the recipes for dietetic lunches and breakfasts-on-the-run. You can't tell these Fat Free Singles are absolutely positively 0 fat and only 5 mg of cholesterol. You'll lose pounds and your heart will thank you.

7. **Are healthy foods more expensive?** Yes, at first glance "healthy" foods (fresh veggies, fat-trimmed chicken, etc.) are more expensive. But factor in what you pay for all those Chitos, Fritos, Doritos, Big Macs and everything else on the junk food list; you'll see that healthy food costs way less than a steady binge diet -- plus not being overweight prevents illness and *medications* to treat illness: cardiovascular disease such as heart attack, heart failure, stroke, kidney failure, peripheral arterial

disease; arthritis in knees and weight-bearing joints; diabetes, blindness and leg amputations from diabetes...want me to continue? How much do those motorized chairs cost? How do you calculate the cost of feeling good, healthy, proud of yourself, and full of renewed energy?

8. Take a break here (whew!) for some **good news**. Even a few pounds lost produces health improvements. Five pounds is a *lot*. Lift, keeping your elbow straight, one of those yellow 5-lb. bags of Domino's sugar. OOF! Heavy, ain't it? Now...*put the package in front of your belly*...and imagine it as awful fat. Surely you can do your belly the favor of losing those five pounds, that Domino's bag of sugar. Or maybe ten pounds (two bags!) or...more? Every bit helps.

9. Why *do* doctors talk most about **belly fat**? Because that paunch is called <u>Central Obesity</u>, and it's worse than fat anywhere else. Arteries and veins from belly fat run directly to the gastrointestinal tract, especially the liver, which is the body's "metabolic engine," the place where cholesterol and sugar are made, stored, and released. Gobs of fat on the belly are constantly gumming this metabolic engine with destructive building blocks which increase blood sugar, bad cholesterol (LDL), and triglycerides, while shutting down production of the good cholesterol (HDL). Increased LDL leads to increased fat deposits inside *all* your arteries -- and narrower arteries means insufficient oxygen supply to your heart & brain, *suffocating them*. Next come heart attacks, strokes, and other trouble. HDL (think of a toilet) helps flush out those fat deposits and returns them to the liver disposal unit.

10. **Go for it Foods:** <u>Vegetables</u>, especially rock stars broccoli and carrots, plus cauliflower and other "cruciferous" yellow, orange, or dark-pigmented veggies which are high in antioxidants. Beans too: pinto, red, black and kidney are filling, low-cal, and terrific sources of antioxidants. **<u>Chicken</u>** (no skin, no fat), **<u>Fish</u>,**

especially salmon and tuna which contain omega-3 fatty acids which help prevent fat deposits in arteries (atherosclerosis). Caveat: only eat twice a week, because of tiny amounts of mercury in it. (Twice a week is ok.) Also: avoid altogether if pregnant or nursing. <u>Fruits</u> (in moderation, they're loaded with sugar), especially those with dark pigmented skins like blueberries & strawberries for their antioxidants. <u>Soy products, tofu:</u> Keep frozen, shelled soybeans (Edamame) in your freezer; add them to soups, stews, anything. And tofu -- buy the firm kind. There's no end of filling, delicious, low-cal recipes using tofu. <u>Olive oil</u>, also canola, sunflower, safflower <u>Nuts</u>: walnuts, pecans, almonds, cashews, peanuts, etc, all are high in beneficial fats (monounsaturated, polyunsaturated) and low in bad fats (saturated). **Walnuts** have become another new rock star. They have omega-3 fatty acids like salmon, and eating a small handful of them daily may help lessen damage-by-fat done to the arteries. A study appearing in late 2006 in the Journal of the American College of Cardiology suggests that walnuts may even have more health benefits than olive oil. Carry a small handful in a Baggie. They're great for snacks. <u>Egg whites</u>: recipes to come for make-ahead breakfasts-on-the-run, lunches, and dinners. <u>Spices</u>: Once you've tasted tarragon-&-garlic recipes, you won't *want* junk food any more. Spices are what make food exciting without the need for fat. Cinnamon, basil, oregano, dill, exotic saffron and ginger... It's fun discovering new recipes, which change depending on how spice is used.

11. **Exercise**: Such a vital, personal subject. See Chapter Six.

12. **Rate of weight loss**: Realistically, two pounds a week, sometimes less. Remember the rabbit and the tortoise. If you try to crash too hard, you'll falter. Try to develop patience. Losing weight in any diet is slow. Accept that. Accept, too, that after the first few days' 3 to 5 pounds of water lost (depending on how high your weight is to begin with), the scale may often read only a pound less in a week. That's okay -- a pound is

a *lot*. Pick up a wrapped pound of meat at the supermarket to see how heavy it is. And persevere. This diet is how you should eat, most of the time, for the rest of your life. The bulk provided by recipes ahead will be satisfying and filling, and the absence of all that sugar will end the insulin highs-and-lows which has you raiding the pantry or McDonald's every 2-3 hours. THAT'S the vicious cycle: *the up-down glucose pattern.* It's easy to break. Just change your whole relationship with food: your glucose pattern will adjust quickly, and last longer.

13. What about "nutrition/diet/meal replacement"/ bars? Um, maybe there's a reason why they taste so good. I bought a bunch the other day. One, sold everywhere, is called a "diet meal replacement bar." It's tiny (2 ounces -- *that's* a meal replacement?), and contains 225 calories including palm oil, butter, and heavy cream equaling 3 grams of saturated fat. The label bears the coy disclaimer "More research is needed to establish a firm relationship between blood sugar and weight control" (duh-h!) and...how many people eat just one!? Read the labels. Another "Nutrition Bar" contains 230 calories, 0 trans fats (ta-dah) -- but 5 grams of saturated fat from Fractionated Palm Oil *(oops! Palm oil's bad)*. These bars are also expensive. Most cost over $2 for a bar weighing under two ounces, which (I'm doing the math) comes out to over twenty dollars a pound. $20 a pound for all that saturated fat! Other "diet bars"...Chocolate Peppermint! Cookies 'n Cream!...you get the idea. Why don't you just buy a Hershey bar? Do people *want* to kid themselves? Read the labels.

14. **Antioxidants** are substances which interfere with the ability of LDL cholesterol to make deposits in the arterial wall. Cocoa is the absolute top antioxidant. Also excellent are those found in highly pigmented foods, such as blueberries, strawberries, red grapes, broccoli, carrots, yellow squash, and zucchini. Dark pigmented is the key. Antioxidants are also in green & black tea, selenium, and Vitamin E. One glass of red wine per day is also

good if there are no contraindications. (Beer on the other hand is produced from grain products and is high in carbohydrates, light beer less so.)

15. **Are some breads okay?** Yes, in moderation: rye, rye with seeds, whole grain wheat, oat and bran, pita and bagels if made with oat bran & whole wheat, Joseph's Oat Bran, Flax, & Whole Wheat Pita (7" wide, delicate like a crepe, 60 calories), and Joseph's Tortillas (8" wide, 70 calories). Great for rollups, diet burritos, and take-to-work lunch. Even "good" carbs metabolize into sugar (more quickly than you think), so go easy on them. Don't drive yourself crazy counting carbs, but be aware.

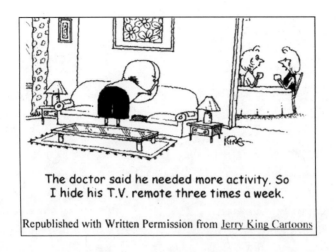

The doctor said he needed more activity. So
I hide his T.V. remote three times a week.

Republished with Written Permission from Jerry King Cartoons

CHAPTER SIX

Exercise

"I joined a health club last year, spent about 400 bucks, haven't
lost a pound. Apparently you have to show up."

Old joke, but it's how most of us feel. Kick boxing? Are you
kidding? What's an elliptical machine? And things like tennis,
swimming, jogging, or Pilates require you to *go* someplace, remake
your life around them, may even be too strenuous for someone just
starting out.

But exercise you must, so here's the magic word: WALK.

Joyce and I have a mini-speedway in our house, and we power-walk
it. (Power walk, apparently, is the new term for what we've been
doing all along.) Twenty-thirty minutes a day, at least five days
a week, we zoom around and around through the kitchen, living
room, front hall, and other rooms back to the kitchen. That's it! If
it meant driving or trudging through the blizzard or July heat to
some gym, we wouldn't do it. We're lazy, prefer climate control.
Does your home or apartment lend itself to a "mini-speedway?"
If there's a room that's a lobster trap (just one door; you can't run
through), could you see having a contractor break through, put a

door in? Years ago we did that to a smaller room. It had one non-support wall blocking the way.

Some people have treadmills, or prefer fast-walking around the block, the neighborhood. Whatever feels best, and works easily into your existing routine. "Sow a habit and reap a destiny." Old saying, applies to exercising too. If you find a routine you can do daily, even if you have to *force yourself* to do it at first, it will soon become a habit. Something, in fact, you'll soon feel guilty about not doing! And proud of yourself when you do do it.

A whole new kind of gratification. Try it. Remember the guy in the London bus, the conductor who had to climb up and down the stairs as opposed to the driver, who just sat.

Thirty minutes of "power walking" (4 mph) uses 225 calories. That's a lot off your daily diet-quota of, say, 1200 or 1300 calories. If you only do twenty minutes a day, fine, but the **weekly tally should amount to 120 minutes.** Two hours a week! That will do the job for you, and you won't hate it. More, say 180 minutes (ten extra minutes a day), will provide slightly more benefit, and fine if you can do it, but it's not enough to knock yourself out for.

Especially if you consider the numbers. The average adult consumes about 2,000 calories per day, and there are approximately 3,500 calories of energy stored in one pound of body fat. So if you eat only 1,200 calories a day, that's a weekly deficit of 5,600, or 1.6 pounds lost. Add to that another 1,400 (burned off in six days' worth of 30 minutes power walks), that's another 0.4 pound of fat lost. On the other hand, if less than 2 pounds lost a week is enough for you, you can up your daily intake by another 100-200 calories a day -- thanks to the exercising! It allows you to eat a bit more without guilt.

Did you know you can also break up your exercise? Do five minutes here, ten minutes there…that's fine, just do it more frequently.

What matters is the day's cumulative amount. Surely you can work in 20 minutes of fast-walking during the day; then there'll just be ten minutes left for after dinner. **Any exercise can be cumulative,** as opposed to sweating it all out all at once.

JUST MOVE MORE, that's the point. If you're waiting before the microwave, instead of just standing there do an in-place step-step-step, a little dance. Have the radio on? *Make the feet move more,* no matter how. Park at the furthest end of the parking lot (if it's daylight, and safe). Take the stairs instead of the elevator (if your health is o.k. for it; check with your physician). If you work on the 30th floor, take the elevator to the 29th floor, and walk the rest. The next week, start walking at the 28th floor, and so on. And…if you're walking from the, ahem, TV to the fridge, take the long way. Then follow your steps *back* to the couch, and repeat. Back and forth, back and forth. Then maybe forget the fridge.

Always check with your doctor before starting any exercise program.

Holding hand weights while you walk uses even more calories. One in each hand -- hup, two, three, four. Bend your elbows slightly as you walk; they'll start to swing with your natural rhythm.

For the psychological and physiologic aspects of dieting and daily life, they're fantastic. Endorphins rule. (Endorphins are peptides produced by the pituitary gland and the hypothalamus; they resemble opiates in their ability to produce analgesia -- painkiller -- and a sense of well-being.)

PART TWO

Food Lists, Meal Plans, and Recipes including
*MLAs
(*make-lots-ahead)

More die in the United States of too much food than of too little. –John K. Galbraith, JFK's Ambassador to India

CHAPTER SEVEN
Food Shopping: Harder Than Before

The good news: You've decided to wean yourself from junk food and eat healthier, home-prepared MLA (Make Lots Ahead) meals. They just involve cooking two or three times a week, which isn't bad, right? (it's Joyce now, back). My credo: cook for a regiment, then freeze, thaw, & reheat. Sound okay? Hooray. Your resolution is made.

Then you go to the supermarket.

Have fun studying the labels. No trans fats! they proclaim, but their Nutrition Facts labels list hydrogenated soybean oil, hydrogenated sunflower oil, on and on. One buttery spread proclaims it's "non-hydrogenated *and* has no trans fats." Guess they think we don't know it's the same thing.

Trans fats are still there. Or if they've taken some out they've replaced it with saturated fat. The FDA guidelines instituted in January of 2006 have failed, because – loophole! -- food manufacturers can actually claim that their product is trans fat-free *as long as it contains less than 1/2 gram (500 mg.) per serving.*[14] Worse, THEY decide what

14   See p. 160: "Reduced-fat" Mayonnaise

a "serving size" is, and make it, like, 1/2 a teaspoon. This labeling trick has allowed trans fats back big time into the stores, fast foods, and your home. "That's extremely disturbing," said Michael D. Ozner, M.D., chairman of the American Heart Association of Miami, "since as few as three daily servings of these supposedly safe foods can increase one's risk of heart disease and diabetes by thirty percent."

According to the USDA, over 42,000 food products on the market still contain trans fats, including forty percent of all prepared foods such as margarines, baking mixes, desserts, spreads, chips, crackers, cereals, and frozen foods.

Be skeptical. If the snazzy package says No Trans Fats, don't automatically believe it and toss it into your cart. Double-check the ingredients for words like "hydrogenated," "partially hydrogenated," or vegetable shortening. (Some have gone back to that old-fashioned term.) "Heart Healthy! 0 trans fat!" says one brand of cracker. But *what's their "serving?" Two crackers?* And if those two crackers add up to 499 mg., which makes it legal to say they have no trans fat, and meanwhile you're happily chowin' 'em down because you think a lot is ok…where does that leave you?

Sicker on the inside. Which isn't even counting the saturated fats -- another artery clogger -- snuck in when they were forced to decrease the trans fats.

Do the math. Count the number of saturated, mono-unsaturated, and poly-unsaturated fat grams on the Nutrition Facts label. If the "Total Fat" number is higher than those three combined, the difference equals what they're hiding. Which is trans fats. The National Academy of Sciences has announced that the only truly safe intake of these harmful fats is zero.

Sneaky ways to beat legislation. Like the nicotine industry's conspiracy that deceived and wrecked people's health for decades.

The upshot is that many people have stopped buying processed foods altogether, and have replaced margarine with canola and olive oil in their recipes. Others are sticking to the outer edges of the grocery store, where the fresh produce, fat free ground turkey, skim milk, yogurt, and eggs are located. Well, maybe duck into a center aisle for some Cheerios or Wheaties or canned good veggies, but that's it. And watch out for "power," "nutrition," and granola bars, they can be loaded with fats and hidden sugars.

Another irony. For years there were many people who didn't cook. But since the trans fat shock, more and more of us are rediscovering our stoves and cookbooks and measuring cups. Because deep down, we know that no food will be as healthy as what we make ourselves. Imagine: home made, no additives! Cooking can also be creative. You study better ways of making things, and then improvise, invent your own recipes. Another thing is that cooking uses up lots of calories. Once I made healthy pizza for family and friends. I was tearing around the kitchen, measuring, pouring, reaching up, stooping down, cleaning...whew! I was sweating! My big surprise was that cooking can also be exercise. Talk about win-win situations.

As for losing weight, remember too that it's a long process. It requires *patience* – just the thing for your instant gratification old self, right? Understand this; accept it. Above all, don't begin with some do-or-die "I gotta lose 20 or 200 pounds" feeling. Rejoice over every pound lost. Your heart will. Your whole body will. You can't see it happening, but it is.

Just remember to *try* not to bring home crackers and snacks, or eat them in the supermarket as you shop, or in the car with the windows rolled up. ☺ If you're hungry, hang in there. Being hungry, ironically, is the thing that *won't* harm you. Also try not to react when you see those big, terrific-looking ads showing Before and After Beauties who lost weight on OUR diet. No they didn't. Or if they did, they put it right back on. "Results aren't typical," admit these ads way down at the bottom of the page in tiny print.

But you're human. As you continue to diet, there will be times when you'll feel yourself weakening, giving second, wistful looks at the scams.

Buy our pill! Lose weight fast and easy! Outta town, call collect! If these worked, WE'd use them. And you'd see nobody fat walking around. And doctors would prescribe them, and we wouldn't have a national obesity epidemic swamping our healthcare system. In your toughest moments, ignore the scams and the ads and appreciate that what you're doing is *hard*. There are no free rides. And you're stronger than you think!

Beware too of: processed "diet" meals in the stores. A recent raid on a local supermarket turned up:

1. A frozen Beef and Broccoli with Noodles "Diet" dinner, whose package (1 serving) read Total fat 14 grams, Saturated fat 4 grams and…surprise…no mention of trans fats. Again, do the math. *What and where are the mystery 10 grams of fat?* If they were "okay" mono- and polyunsaturated fats, they'd say so. This meal also contained (ugh) 34 grams of carbs and 9 grams of sugar. For…one…serving. Other pre-cooked frozen "diet" meals with names like HEALTHY THIS and FIT LIFE THAT turned out just as bad. Again, read the labels. Judge for yourself.

2. "Low Fat Waffles," unfortunately, were loaded with carbs (38 grams) and sugar (6 grams). Too much. I'll teach you to make OK pancakes & waffles. They're easy.

3. A No-Sugar Fudge Topping, sad to say, contained 24 grams of carbs in just 1 1/2 tablespoons -- and who eats just 1 1/2 tablespoons? This product is fattening!

No rice, pasta, or couscous here

Carbs-wise, couscous is the same as rice, corn, & regular pasta. This program has enough carbs from fruits, veggies, healthy pitas, and cereals. More would be bad. Carbs alone can cause overweight and diabetes. *Exception: <u>Shirataki tofu noodles and fettuccini</u>, *1/30th the carbs* as regular noodles. As of this writing they're only available at Gristede's, Trader Joe's, and online from Amazon.com. The manufacturer is House Foods America Corporation, house-foods. com. (They have a taste which isn't quite that of regular pasta. But they're filling for fast weight loss.)

Also <u>Dreamfields</u> Low Carb Pastas: taste the same as regular pasta, but have *1/8th the carbs*. Also more shapes such as lasagna, rotini, penne, linguini, & elbows. They're becoming widely available, but you can also order them from dreamfieldsfoods.com or amazon. com/Dreamfields

• • •

What about Chinese Take-Out?

Stir-Fry Vegetables is filling and low in fat/sugar/calories. Ditto chicken and snow peas, or shrimp and broccoli (275 calories per serving) -- entrees that are fine. You can eat out or take out. But -- no egg rolls, spare ribs...you know which ones are okay. Substitute the good ones for any lunch or dinner.

This Diet's Meals are also Mix and Match

Switch around the breakfasts, lunches, and dinners ahead any way you like, the calories are all counted for you. (Just keep track. Got a calculator?) Many *Make Lots Ahead breakfasts can also double as any-time snacks. Picture delicate pita, soaked first in egg whites, then sautéed in hot olive oil. Make a stack of 'em and freeze. Do the same with rye bread or whole wheat bagels. Grab 'em and run in the morning.

Keep an OxBox Too

What's an OxBox? It's just a plastic fridge container full of fresh broccoli florets & already-peeled small carrots -- the most anti-oxidant-intense veggies full of fiber. We munch on them often. And having them already there, in that cellophane-covered box, is as easy as sticking your hand into a bag of Something Bad. The impulse thing we all do. Just substitute the habit.

Tomorrow, you begin, and *don't forget to exercise! Walk 5 minutes here, 5 minutes there, 10 or 15 minutes after dinner…but get it up to 30 minutes a day. Gotta flush those arteries!*

On the next page you'll find the list of Healthy New Products to help you get thin.

Hang in there…and Good Luck!

GREAT NEW PRODUCTS FOR DIET AND HEALTH

"My life, my joy, my food …!" – Shakespeare, *King John (act III, sc. IV, line 103)*

We shouldn't blame ourselves, or the "American diet." People have always loved food, but unless they were rich they didn't have much. Probably if junk food existed 100 years ago, our history books's photos would have been full of fat people. We're human.

But the abundance is now a tsunami, and the main culprit is sugar. The average American consumes *142 pounds of sugar per year*, up from 100 pounds 30 years ago Most of what we eat is either sugar or metabolizes faster than you think into sugar -- and from there into artery-clogging, diabetes-and-cancer-causing F-A-T. So let's start with artificial sweeteners, most of which are quite safe. (See p. 25-26.) From there we'll move on to other New Products for Diet and Health.

Splenda: contains 1% sucralose, which is itself FDA-approved. 0 calories, 0 total fat, less than 1 g carb, 0 cholesterol. Works best in beverages and baking, but lacks the binding power (can't make the cookie stiff) of real sugar. In every baking recipe you can just replace *half* the sugar requirement with Splenda. For structure, volume, & height, Splenda recipes will tell you to add honey, brown sugar, molasses and maple syrup. Hello? They're all pure sugar. Home/online recipes will suggest agave, chopped dates, condensed juices, fat free evaporated milk (45 g carbs in a 12 oz can =11 tsp sugar). Same thing. Sugar just as real as the white stuff in a sugar bowl. Splenda's still a boon, though. Just be aware.

Aspartame: Same good news. Aspartame (Equal, Nutrataste) is great in your coffee, all beverages, and sells in Diet Coke and practically everything else. Both Splenda and Aspartame have decades-long track records and many studies in humans: no red flags, as physicians say.

<u>100% Liquid Egg Whites</u>: 3 tablespoons=1 egg, 25 calories, 0 total fat, 0 mg cholesterol, 0 g sugar. Tops for avoiding artery-clogging yolks, whipping up all kinds of meals a day, plus using for baking.

<u>Ener-G Egg Replacer</u>: Ditto above. Good if recipe calls for two or more yolks. If one only yolk is required (meaning it's only needed for binding), you can also use 1 heaping tablespoon baking powder, 1 heaping tablespoon olive oil, plus 1 tablespoon warm water.

<u>Fat Free Cheddar & American Cheese</u>, shredded or Singles: each slice 30 calories, 0 total fat, less than 5 mg cholesterol, 1 g sugar, 5 g protein. Use with eggs, baking, everything.

<u>Fat Free Mozarella</u>, shredded or Singles: In 1 oz slice, 35 calories, 0 total fat, less than 5 mg cholesterol, 1 g carb, less than 1 g sugar. Great for ziti, lasagna, sliced with tomatoes, everything. Try this sandwich: 2 slices rye with seeds, Dijon mustard, sliced fat free mozzarella, & tomatoes. (& fresh basil leaves if you can get them)

<u>Fat Free Sour Cream</u>: in 2 tablespoons 30 calories, 0 total fat, less than 5 mg cholesterol, 2 g sugar

<u>Fat Free Cream Cheese</u>, 0 fat, 1 g carb, 15 calories per 2 tablespoons. Everything from cheese cake to no-fat, elegant Nova Scotia & cream cheese dip, or smear 1 tbsp on toasted rye with seeds: Yum.

<u>Fat Free Ricotta Cheese</u>: in 1/4 cup 40 calories, 0 total fat, 15 mg cholesterol, 3 g sugar

<u>Fat Free whipped topping</u>: in 2 tablespoons 15 calories, 0 total fat, 0 cholesterol, 1g sugar. Fun, festive, & zero-guilt.

<u>Shirataki tofu noodles and fettuccini</u>, *1/30th* the carbs of regular pasta! – plus there's evidence that they may have other health benefits, such as lowering cholesterol and blood sugar. It comes packaged in cool liquid, is stored in refrigerator sections next to tofu, and you must rinse off its liquid, then par-boil. Available at house-foods.com, Amazon.com, or Trader Joe's.

<u>Dreamfields Low Carb Pasta</u>, 1/8th the carbs. Offers lasagna, linguini, penne, elbows, & rotini. All 0 total fat, 0 cholesterol. It's excellent. Here's their blurb: "A typical 2-oz serving of regular pasta is an astounding 42g carbs, but Dreamfields pasta has only 5g digestible carbs, and helps limit by 65% the rise in blood glucose levels that normally occur after eating ordinary pasta. Should be available at most stores or health stores, or dreamfieldsfoods.com or Amazon.

<u>Log Cabin Sugar Free Maple Syrup</u>: 35 calories per 1/4 cup, 0 total fat, 0 cholesterol, 12 g sugar (from sugar alcohol). This is so good we've thrown out our regular, pure-sugar maple syrup.

Milled Flax Seed: Recommended dose: two tablespoons a day. May be one of the most powerful natural cholesterol controllers (its Omega-3 oils push down LDL). Use in pancakes, baked goods, sprinkle on cereal, salads, anything. *Milled flax seed can also replace oil & fat at a ratio of 3 to 1.* (3 tbsp. = 1 tbsp butter, margarine, or oil, for ex.) Regular flax seed does not have the benefits of milled flax seed.

<u>Whole Grain Soy Flour</u>: 35 % protein, gluten-free. Use for muffins, pancakes; also to thicken gravies & sauces. In 1/4 cup, 120 calories, 6 g fat (1 g saturated), 0 mg cholesterol, 8 g carbs (3 g dietary fiber), 2 g sugar, 10 g protein. A hamburger has 12 grams protein. * In any recipe calling for all-purpose flour, replace 1/3 (or slightly less) of it with soy flour. Since soy flour has no gluten, which gives structure to yeast-raised breads, it can't replace all the wheat flour. Also, it's a little bitter; you may want to add some Splenda.

* Baking with soy flour may brown more quickly. Try reducing baking time or lower oven temperature slightly.
* Use soy flour as a cholesterol-free egg substitute in baked goods. Replace one egg with one tablespoon soy flour and one tablespoon water.

(Bobsredmill.com, HodgsonMill.com)

SOY PROTEIN POWDER: I'm wild about this; am still trying to figure ways to put it in everything. Different from Soy Flour, it's fluffy and sweet; 1/3 cup soy powder packs in 24 grams of protein, equal to two hamburgers. Use it in Smoothies, mix it in your yogurt, replace up to half the flour in many baking recipes. The FDA says that 25 g. of soy protein daily helps reduce the risk of heart disease & helps lower LDL cholesterol. (Just beware of "power bars" & commericial Smoothies that contain sugar, in any form.)

Whole Wheat Pastry Flour: better taste & high nutritional value. All whole grain natural fiber, original oils & vitamins. 1/4 cup = 100 calories, total fat .5 mg (0 saturated fat), 0 mg cholesterol, 3 g protein total carbohydrate 22 g (dietary fiber 4 g).

Joseph's Pita & Tortillas: made with flax, oat bran & whole wheat. They're more delicate, like crepes. Their pita pockets are 60 calories & have just 1.5 grams fat, 0 cholesterol, 5g dietary fiber, 1 g sugar, and 7 g protein. Good for meals-on-the-run.

Sugar Free Tang: all the goodness of o.j., which is otherwise also loaded with sugar.

Minute Maid Just 10 Fruit Punch: A good sugar-removed lunch or take-to-work beverage in a pouch. Good source of calcium & fortified with 100% of the daily value of vitamin C. 10 calories, 2 g sugar per pouch: 90% less sugar than "real" orange juice, apple juice etc.

Diet Beverages: (antioxidant Vitamin C without the calories)
*Crystal Light Ready to Serve, 5 calories per 8 oz, flavors include Fruit Punch, Raspberry Lemonade, Iced Tea, Peach Tea, Lemonade, Sunrise Orange, Pineapple/Orange, others

*Ocean Spray Light: 40 calories (5 flavors)
*Ocean Spray Diet Juice Drinks: 5 calories (2 flavors)

<u>Jell-O Sugar-Free Fat-Free Pudding & Gelatins</u>: This product has made dessert fun again, & is used A LOT in this diet. Pudding flavors: Chocolate, Cheesecake, Vanilla, Lemon, Banana Cream, Fudge. Gelatin flavors: Orange, Black Cherry, Lime, Strawberry, Raspberry, Cherry, & more. All puddings, if made with fat-free milk, have per 1/2 cup 70 calories, 0 g total fat, 0 g carbs, 6 g carbs (from the milk). Excellent product. Make all kinds of desserts. For toppings: try plain fat-free yogurt mixed with artificial sweetener, then mixed with 1 tsp of any Jello flavor, then sprinkled with walnuts, strawberries, blueberries, this diet's chocolate sauce & fat free whipped topping, etc. Yum! No guilt! No kidding!

<u>Athens Fillo (Phyllo) Dough and Mini Fillo Shells</u>: 0 total fat, 0 cholesterol, 0-2 g sugar. (Minis are 18 calories each.) Great for crusts and everything from appetizers to quiche, strudel, and pizza.

<u>Sugar Free Jams & Preserves</u>: Great for baking, cooking, even spread on something healthy with your No Fat Cream Cheese.

* <u>Polaner</u> Sugar Free Preserves all have **10** calories per tablespoon, 0 total fat, 0 sugar (5g total carbs – the fruit) Their flavors are: Strawberry, Apricot, Concord Grape Jelly, Orange Marmalade, Seedless Raspberry, Seedless Blackberry, Pineapple, Blueberry, Black Cherry, Peach, & Mint.

* <u>Smuckers</u> also has Apricot, Blueberry, Grape, Orange Marmalade, Peach, Raspberry, Strawberry & others, all made with Splenda. Nutritional info the same: **10** calories per tablespoon, Total fat 0 g, Total Carbs 5 g (the fruit), sugar 0g.

<u>Whole Grain Breads</u>: Bear in mind that the "good carbs" of healthy bread are still carbs which break down to sugar. More slowly, true, but it's still important to know if you're diabetic or pre-diabetic.

Important Regular Staples

Small & lg. plastic fridge containers

Silicone-coated Parchment Paper (no greasing needed, best for baking)

Nut Chopper (with grind handle & lid)

Splenda

Equal

Unsweetened Cocoa (Natural, non-alkanized; Hershey's is good)

Pure Vanilla Extract

Non-fat milk (with lactose-free you can do dessert tricks)

Eggs, fresh

Liquid egg whites

Cream of Tartar (1/4 tsp per 2 egg whites adds stability in meringues & soufflés)

Fat-Free cheese slices (Kraft is excellent)

Yogurt, fat free

Tofu, extra firm

Strawberries & blueberries (frozen ok; nutrients not affected)

Apples

Carrots, small already-peeled kind

Fresh & frozen broccoli

Cauliflower, frozen

Fresh Peppers, red, yellow, orange (wash, cut, and store frozen in a Ziploc)

Frozen shelled soybeans (Edamame)

Onions, fresh

Chicken breasts or tenderloins, frozen (trim all fat; freeze)

Ground turkey, fat free (ok to freeze)

Tuna, 7 oz. Cans

Beans, canned: pinto, red, black and kidney

Dijon mustard
Red wine vinegar
Balsamic vinegar
Olive oil (extra virgin)

Walnuts, lightly salted almonds, pecans (See p. 11: walnuts may have even more health benefits than olive oil. Carry a handful in a Baggie; great for snack attacks) All nuts have "good" mono- & polyunsaturated fats. Almonds have twice the calcium of walnuts, & nearly half your daily need of vitamin E, an anti-oxidant that helps boost your immune system. But walnuts have more than your daily need for omega-3 fatty acids, which help lower your triglyceride levels. They're delicious, though, and have 10 calories per nut. Don't overdo it.

Bread: rye, rye with seeds, whole wheat, oat and bran, *pita and bagels (oat bran & whole wheat) Joseph's Oat Bran & Whole Wheat Pita (7" wide, delicate & sweeter like a crepe, only 60 calories); Joseph's Oat Bran & Whole Wheat Tortillas (8" wide, 70 calories)... great to fill or for rollups, diet burritos, take-to-work lunch

Spices: garlic, tarragon, cinnamon, pepper, basil, oregano, dill, ginger
Tomato paste
Sun-dried tomatoes in jars with olive oil
Barbecue Sauce
Chicken broth, fat-free, no sodium
Soups: Fat free Minestrone, Lentil

Sugar substitute: Equal, NatraTaste, Splenda (all totally safe; no processed-fructose-type adverse affects)

Diet sodas (ok if made with Splenda, Aspartame)

This is a list of basic non-perishables. Recipes will also call for fresh dairy and produce.

DAILY MEAL PLANS
Update in Nutrition and Cardiology

Day 1*

*Each recipe's calories are tallied, so if you find favorites you can switch around & still keep track.

<u>Breakfast</u>
MLA New Age Pancake... 112 calories
Sprinkle with either cinnamon[15] or unsweetened cocoa mixed with equal parts artificial sweetener. Or Sugar-Free maple syrup, 1/4 c
.... 35 calories
Coffee with nonfat milk and artificial sweetener......... 10 calories

<u>Lunch</u>
Turkey rollup .... 212 calories
Berry Intense Smoothie... 75 calories

<u>Midafternoon Snack</u>
2 tbsp Fudge Sauce on 4 oz nonfat yogurt mixed with 1 tsp powder of Sugar-Free Orange Jello.. 100 calories

<u>Dinner</u>
4 oz MLA Chicken Marsala....................................... 250 calories
Diet Coke

<u>Dessert</u>
Chocolate Ice Cream with whipped topping .... 85 calories
Cappuccino with Cinnamon .... 10 calories

<u>Evening snack</u>
5 walnuts, 5 almonds, & 1/2 cup seedless red grapes 150 calories
Hot Cocoa .... 40 calories

Total: 1079

Unsweetened cocoa acts like a mood altering drug (relaxing artery walls, increasing a sense of optimism) that will help you to stay feeling good.

---

15 Besides having powerful antioxidants, cinnamon in doses as low as 1/2 tea-spoon daily significantly reduces blood sugar, triglycerides, and LDL-choles-terol (L for Lousy)

Day 2*

*Check that your unsweetened cocoa is natural, non-alkalinized. Alkanization, or "Dutch processed," destroys the antioxidants.

<u>Breakfast</u>
MLA Banana Muffin... 120 calories
(typical of this diet's new way to bake: Splenda, no bad flour, no yolks. In this one case, some sugar in the form of ripened banana.)
Coffee with skim milk & sugar substitute................. 10 calories

<u>Lunch</u>
Quiche .... 158 calories
Green tea with artificial sweetener

<u>Midafternoon snack</u>
Chocolate Smoothie .... 90 calories
5 walnuts & 5 almonds... 100 calories

<u>Dinner</u>
4 oz Salmon Dijon .... 265 calories
Crudités with MLA Vinaigrette............................... 125 calories

<u>Dessert</u>
Chocolate Mousse (Luscious, no-fat, no-sugar!) .... 100 calories
Cappuccino with Cinnamon .... 10 calories

<u>Evening snack</u>
1 Joseph's pita .... 60 calories
2 Tbsp Philadelphia Fat-Free Cream Cheese .... 30 calories
1 tbsp Strawberry Sugar Free Preserves .... 10 calories

Total: 1078

What exactly *is* a hunger pang? It's a brief muscular spasm. Like an itch, if you tough it out, it will pass.

Day 3

Breakfast
Scrambled eggs & cheese in pita .... 135 calories
Hot cocoa .... 40 calories

Lunch
Tuna Salad with Mayonnaise substitute .... 167 calories
Strawberry Smoothie .... 90 calories

Midafternoon Snack
2 tbsp Fudge Sauce on 4 oz nonfat yogurt mixed with 1 tsp powder
of Black Cherry Jello & 1/2 cup red seedless grapes.. 150 calories

Dinner
4 oz MLA Tex Mex Chicken .... 215 calories
*save leftovers for tomorrow's lunch

Dessert
3 Fudge Nut Tarts.. 105 calories
Cappuccino with Cinnamon .... 10 calories

Evening snack
Anytime Blondie.. 169 calories
Sugar Free Tang*.. 5 calories
*Difference between vitamin-enriched above & "real" o.j.: 24 grams
sugar, which equals 6 tsp table sugar (divide by 4)

Total:...1086

**Uncomfortable fact: Norwegians were actually healthier
during the brutal Nazi occupation, when everyone starved. At
war's end their diabetes, strokes, and heart attacks spiked...**

Day 4

Breakfast
Anytime Cheese 'n Onions Bar TM .... 112 calories
Mocha Latte.. 100 calories

Lunch
3 oz *MLA Tex Mex chicken .... 161 calories
Green tea with sugar substitute

Midafternoon snack
3 Chocolate Candies broken up into 4 oz nonfat yogurt mixed with
1 tsp powder of Lime Jello... 80 calories

Dinner
Fettucini Alfredo .... 320 calories
(1/30 the carbs of regular pasta)

Dessert
Vanilla Ice Cream, Fudge Sauce & whipped topping 125 calories
Cappuccino with Cinnamon .... 10 calories

Evening snack
New Age Brownie .... 97 calories
Crystal Light Raspberry Lemonade .... 5 calories

Total:..1014

Most diets fail because of boredom & impatience, not hunger.

Day 5

<u>Breakfast</u>
Anytime Brownie .... 185 calories
Coffee with nonfat milk and sugar substitute .... 10 calories

<u>Lunch</u>
MLA Western Omelet .... 215 calories
Chocolate Drink (cool or hot) ....40 calories

<u>Midafternoon snack</u>
2 tbsp fudge sauce on 1 tsp powdered Jello Vanilla Pudding & 1/2
cup drained mandarin oranges mixed in 4 oz nonfat yogurt ....
.... 150 calories

<u>Dinner</u>
MLA Lemon-Garlic Marinated Shrimp .... 100 calories
2 oz. Shirataki noodles... 10 calories
(Available locally, Amazon.com, or www.house-foods.com)

<u>Dessert</u>
Cheesecake with strawberries & fudge sauce............. 188 calories

<u>Evening snack</u>
5 walnuts, 5 almonds, & 1/2 cup seedless red grapes..................
.... 150 calories

Total..1048

**Food idea rejected by MacDonalds: Way Too Damn Happy
Meal**

Day 6

<u>Breakfast</u>
Quiche .... 158 calories
Coffee with nonfat milk and sugar substitute .... 10 calories

<u>Lunch</u>
Stir-Fry vegetables (Take-Out or make it) .... 225 calories
Green tea with sugar substitute

<u>Midafternoon snack</u>
5 walnuts, 5 almonds, 1/2 cup seedless grapes .... 150 calories
Hot Cocoa .... 40 calories

<u>Dinner</u>
Tuna Vinaigrette , 4 oz .... 320 calories
Diet Sprite

<u>Dessert</u>
Pear, Pudding & Chocolate Sauce .... 115 calories
Cappuccino.. 10 calories

<u>Evening snack</u>
3 cups plain popcorn .... 25 calories
Minute Maid Just 10 vitamin fortified fruit drink ..... 10 calories

Total:...1063

Tom Hanks, playing Jimmy Dugan in **A LEAGUE OF THEIR OWN**: "It's *supposed* to be hard. If it wasn't hard, everyone would do it. The *hard* is what *makes* it great."

Day 7

Breakfast
2 MLA Pita Pancakes.................................. 173 calories
Sprinkle with either cinnamon or unsweetened cocoa mixed with
equal parts artificial sweetener.
Coffee with nonfat milk and sugar substitute............. 10 calories

Lunch
Rye & Cheese sandwich .... 270 calories

Midafternoon snack
2 tbsp fudge sauce on 4 oz nonfat yogurt mixed with1 tsp powder
Orange Sugar-Free Jello & 1/2 cup strawberries .... 150 calories

Dinner
4 oz Chicken Cacciatore .... 245 calories
(Make extra for day 9)

Dessert
Apple Crisp with whipped topping .... 118 calories
Cappuccino... 10 calories

Evening snack
1 Joseph's pita, 2 tbsp Fat Free Cream Cheese............ 90 calories

Total: 1066

Avoid weighing yourself too often. This becomes compulsive
& heightens impatience. Once or twice a week is ok.

Day 8

Breakfast
Anytime Cheese & Turkey Bar™ .... 163 calories
Coffee or tea with skim milk and sugar substitute ..... 10 calories

Lunch
Tuna Melt rollup .... 255 calories
Green tea with sugar substitute

Midafternoon snack
Chocolate Smoothie .... 90 calories

Dinner
Linguine with White Clam Sauce .... 335 calories
Diet Sprite

Dessert
Fruit Chocolate Fondue .... 140 calories
Cappuccino.. 10 calories

Evening snack
1 pita & 2 tbsp fat free cream cheese .... 90 calories

Total:...1093

Seventh Day Adventists are vegetarians. They have the lowest rate of coronary disease in America.

Day 9

Breakfast
Tomato & cheese Pita .... 160 calories

Lunch
3 oz Chicken Cacciatore... 206 calories
Green tea with sugar substitute

Midafternoon snack
1 medium-sized banana & 4 oz nonfat yogurt sweetened with 1 tsp
Jello Orange & 2 tbsp fudge sauce .... 170 calories
Ocean Spray Orange Citrus Drink .... 5 calories

Dinner
4 oz MLA Chicken Tarragon with grapes & walnuts 255 calories
(save extra for tomorrow's lunch)

Dessert
Chocolate Berry Parfait... 125 calories
Cappuccino... 10 calories

Evening snack
1 toasted rye with seeds & 1/4 cup no-fat cottage cheese
.... 130 calories

Total 1061

Keep a diary. Under lock & key if necessary. Write how you're doing and feeling, & not just with the diet. So much eating comes from boredom or emotions. Eating helps neither; writing is a constructive outlet for both. Tap into your creativity. Let it rip.

Day 10

Breakfast
Anytime Cheese 'n Onions Bar .... 112 calories
Mocha Latte... 100 calories

Lunch
*3 oz MLA Chicken Tarragon with grapes .... 185 calories
Chocolate drink, hot or cold .... 40 calories

Midafternoon snack
5 walnuts & 5 almonds .... 100 calories
Berry Intense Smoothie.. 75 calories

Dinner
Nova Scotia omelet... 225 calories

Dessert
Chocolate pudding with strawberries......................... 93 calories
Cappuccino .... 10 calories

Evening snack
Whole Wheat Mini Bagel .... 100 calories
2 Tbsp Philadelphia Fat-Free Cream Cheese .... 30 calories

Total:...1070

Think thin. Look at that cake or junk food and imagine how you'll feel *after* you eat it, not while.

Day 11

Breakfast
Anytime Blondie .... 169 calories
Coffee or tea with nonfat milk and sugar substitute ... 10 calories

Lunch
Cheese and Veggies Pita Pocket .... 200 calories
Green tea with sugar substitute

Midafternoon snack
2 tbsp Fudge Sauce on 4 oz nonfat yogurt mixed with 1 tsp sugar
free Jello Chocolate Pudding & 1/2 cup blueberries . 150 calories
Sugar Free Tang .... 5 calories

Dinner
Spaghetti & *MLA meatballs................................... 260 calories
*refrigerate meatballs for future lunch

Dessert
Orange Walnut Mousse with Fudge Sauce .... 120 calories
Cappuccino.. 10 calories

Evening snack
Apple muffin .... 130 calories
Crystal Light Raspberry Lemonade .... 5 calories

Total: 1059

NOTHING TASTES AS GOOD AS BEING THIN FEELS

Day 12

Breakfast
MLA New Age Pancake .... 112 calories
Log Cabin Sugar Free maple syrup, 1/4 cup .... 35 calories
Coffee with nonfat milk and sugar substitute

Lunch
3 meatballs.. 155 calories
1 pita with a little sauce .... 70 calories
Diet Coke

Midafternoon snack
1/2 cup seedless red grapes, 5 almonds, 5 walnuts.... 150 calories
Hot or Cold Chocolate Drink .... 40 calories

Dinner
Polynesian Chicken .... 215 calories

Dessert
Lemon Mousse with Fudge Sauce .... 100 calories
Cappuccino... 10 calories

Evening snack
1 toasted rye slice with seeds & 1/4 cup no-fat cottage cheese
.... 130 calories

Total:..1047

Resolve weakening? Picture someone saying, "Oh, you look so thin!!"

Day 13

Breakfast
Anytime Cheese & Onions Bar .... 112 calories
Coffee with nonfat milk and sugar substitute............. 10 calories

Lunch
Rye & Cheese Sandwich... 270 calories
Green tea with sugar substitute

Midafternoon snack
1/2 cup blueberries & 1 tbsp Black Cherry sugar-free Jello mixed in
4 oz nonfat yogurt .... 110 calories
Chocolate Drink .... 40 calories

Dinner
MLA *Chilli, 4 oz .... 210 calories

Dessert
New Age Brownie .... 102 calories
2 tbsp fudge sauce & 2 tbsp fat free whipped topping
.... 55 calories

Evening snack
Banana Oatmeal Muffin... 120 calories
Ocean Spray Cranberry Drink....................................... 5 calories

Total: 1034

*That 28 oz can of Crushed Tomatoes you'll use for this recipe?
Keep your elbow straight and heft it your hand. Heaaavy!
You'll say, "I've lost more than *this*?" Yep. And your blood
sugar's dropping...

Day 14

<u>Breakfast</u>
Anytime Brownie .... 185 calories
Coffee with non fat milk.. 10 calories

<u>Lunch</u>
Cheese and Veggies Pita Pocket.............................. 200 calories
Green tea with sugar substitute

<u>Midafternoon snack</u>
5 almonds, 5 walnuts, & 1/2 cup dried apricots .... 150 calories
Ocean Spray Orange Citrus Drink .... 5 calories

<u>Dinner</u>
Garlic shrimp & Vegetables...................................... 275 calories

<u>Dessert</u>
Chocolate Mousse topped with strawberries .... 125 calories
Cappuccino with Cinnamon .... 10 calories

<u>Evening snack</u>
2 Tbsp Philadelphia Fat-Free Cream Cheese .... 30 calories
1 pita... 60 calories
fresh tomato slices .... 5 calories

Total:..1055

Overheard in an elevator: "I feel virtuous when I'm hungry."

Day 15

Breakfast
2 MLA Pita Pancakes.. 174 calories
Sprinkle with either cinnamon or unsweetened cocoa mixed with equal parts artificial sweetener. Or pour on 1/4 cup Log Cabin Sugar-Free maple syrup .... 35 calories
Coffee with nonfat milk and sugar substitute............. 10 calories

Lunch
Turkey rollup .... 215 calories
Green tea with sugar substitute

Midafternoon snack
1/2 cup blueberries in 4 oz nonfat yogurt mixed with 1 tbsp unsweetened cocoa & 1 tbsp Splenda .... 120 calories
Mocha Latte.. 100 calories

Dinner
4 oz MLA Chicken Stroganoff.................................. 235 calories
(Set some aside for tomorrow's lunch; freeze extra)

Dessert
Chocolate Ice Cream with Fudge Sauce & Whipped Topping
.... 125 calories
Decaf Coffee

Evening snack
3 cups plain popcorn, no butter, no salt .... 25 calories
Minute Maid Just 10 vitamin fortified fruit drink ..... 10 calories

Total:...1049

If you are what you eat, I eat broccoli. Does that make me broccoli?

Day 16

<u>Breakfast</u>
Quiche .... 158 calories
Hot Cocoa .... 40 calories

<u>Lunch</u>
3 oz MLA Chicken Stroganoff................................. 176 calories
Berry Intense Smoothie... 75 calories

<u>Midafternoon snack</u>
Chocolate Smoothie with fat free whipped topping.. 115 calories

<u>Dinner</u>
4 oz MLA Lasagna .... 325 calories
(save some for tomorrow's lunch)
1/2 cup green beans sautéed with garlic..................... 25 calories

<u>Dessert</u>
Apple Crisp with whipped topping .... 118 calories
Cappuccino.. 10 calories

<u>Evening snack</u>
3 cups plain popcorn .... 25 calories
Diet Soda

Total:...1067

A diet is the penalty we pay for exceeding the feed limit.

Day 17

Breakfast
Banana Oatmeal Muffin.. 120 calories
Coffee or tea with skim milk and sugar substitute ..... 10 calories

Lunch
3 oz MLA Lasagna .... 244 calories
Chocolate Drink .... 40 calories

Midafternoon snack
1/2 cup seedless red grapes, 5 almonds, 5 walnuts.... 150 calories

Dinner
*MLA Shrimp Scampi .... 215 calories.
2 oz Tofu *Shirataki* Noodles: .... 20 calories.
(Dreamfields would be 190 calories per 2 oz. Serving)

Dessert
New Age Brownie .... 102 calories
2 tbsp fat free whipped topping................................ 15 calories
2 tbsp fudge sauce .... 40 calories

Evening snack
1 toasted rye with seeds & 1/4 cup no-fat cottage cheese
.... 130 calories

Total:..1086

"Health food makes me sick." -- Calvin Trillin

Day 18

Breakfast
Anytime Cheese 'n Onions Bar .... 112 calories
Mocha Latte... 100 calories

Lunch
Stir-Fry vegetables .... 226 calories
Minute Maid 'Just 10' vitamin fortified fruit drink.... 10 calories

Midafternoon snack
1/2 cup blueberries in 4 oz nonfat yogurt mixed with 1 tbsp
unsweetened cocoa & 1 tbsp Splenda .... 120 calories
Sugar Free Tang... 5 calories

Dinner
4 oz Chicken Parmigiana... 253 calories
(save some for Day 20's lunch)

Dessert
Fruit Chocolate Fondue .... 140 calories
Cappuccino... 10 calories

Evening snack
2 Mini-quiches .... 90 calories
Crystal Light Raspberry Lemonade .... 5 calories

Total:...1071

Sign you'll never see: **CARROT-EATERS ANONYMOUS DISBANDED**

Day 19

Breakfast
Scrambled eggs & cheese pita .... 135 calories
Coffee with nonfat milk and sugar substitute............. 10 calories

Lunch
Turkey Rollup .... 212 calories
Ocean Spray Cranberry Drink.................................... 5 calories

Midafternoon snack
Berry Intense Smoothie.. 75 calories
5 walnuts, 5 almonds .... 100 calories

Dinner
4 oz Penne Rigate with Chicken & Broccoli............. 340 calories

Dessert
Lime & Chocolate Dazzler .... 110 calories
Cappuccino .... 10 calories

Evening snack
1 Joseph's Pita... 60 calories
1 Tbsp Philadelphia Fat-Free Cream Cheese .... 15 calories

Total:...1072

Seven days without chocolate makes one weak.

Day 20

<u>Breakfast</u>
Banana Muffin .... 120 calories
Coffee with nonfat milk and sugar substitute............ 10 calories

<u>Lunch</u>
3 oz MLA Chicken Parmigiana............................... 190 calories
Minute Maid 'Just 10' vitamin fortified fruit drink.... 10 calories

<u>Midafternoon snack</u>
Anytime Blondie... 169 calories
Hot cocoa... 40 calories

<u>Dinner</u>
Quiche .... 158 calories
Crudites drizzled with Vinaigrette.......................... 200 calories

<u>Dessert</u>
Chocolate Mousse .... 100 calories
Cappuccino... 10 calories

<u>Evening snack</u>
3 cups plain popcorn .... 25 calories
Minute Maid Just 10 vitamin fortified fruit drink ..... 10 calories

Total:..1042

Being overweight is no weigh to live.

Day 21

<u>Breakfast</u>
Anytime Brownie .... 185 calories
Strawberry Smoothie .... 90 calories

<u>Lunch</u>
Turkey & Cheese Bar .... 163 calories
Diet Coke

<u>Midafternoon snack</u>
3 Chocolate Candies broken up into 4 oz non-fat yogurt mixed
with 1 tsp sugar free Blackberry Jello, 1/2 cup blueberries
.... 130 calories

<u>Dinner</u>
MLA Chicken Tarragon with grapes & walnuts........ 255 calories

<u>Dessert</u>
Vanilla pudding, fudge sauce & whipped topping.... 125 calories
Cappuccino.. 10 calories

<u>Evening snack</u>
Apple muffin .... 130 calories
Crystal Light Raspberry Lemonade .... 5 calories

Total:...1093

**Calvin Trillin spoke lovingly of his wife who had "a weird
predilection for limiting our family to three meals a day"**

RECIPES: *Breakfasts/Lunches/Snacks*

MLA *Pita Pancake*
recipe below for 3, 87 calories each

Cooking spray
3 pitas .... 60 ea.
1/2 cup liquid egg whites .... 60 c.
1/4 cup fat free milk .... 20 c.

Spray skillet with cooking spray. Mix egg whites & milk in bowl.
Soak pita in egg & milk 2 minutes, turning once for more
absorption. (Or tear pita into pieces, soak, then cook. This creates
a thicker pancake.) Grill on medium high heat until brown; turn
& brown other side

Total for 3 pancake pitas: 260 calories, or **87 calories** each.
If you have the time for a more leisurely breakfast: <u>Log Cabin
Sugar Free Maple Syrup</u> has only **35** calories per 1/4 cup, with
0 total fat & 12 g of sugar alcohol. And <u>Philadelphia Fat Free
Cream Cheese</u> has only **15** calories per tablespoon. It's delicious,
with 0 total fat, .5 mg cholesterol, & 1 g carb.

*Hot Cocoa, Chocolate Drink

Mix together two tablespoons Unsweetened Cocoa (40 calories) &
2 tbsp artificial sweetener. Stir with *water hot or cold. That's all.

Fun idea: keep a container full in fridge, ready to just shake
well and pour. For any size: equal amounts cocoa and artificial
sweetener, then water, that's all. **Hot Cocoa with fat free
whipped topping** adds only 15 calories per drink. Total: 55
calories.

*There's evidence that milk inhibits the absorption of flavanols, &
you'll get plenty of protein and calcium from other sources.

MLA New Age Pancakes: Google "no sugar, low carb pancake; searched "big" diet sites and books too. Ads were the usual: **Lose Weight Fast! No Sugar Added!** And they contain…

- 1/2 cup all-purpose flour (metabolizes almost as fast as sugar)
- 2 tablespoons brown sugar (Guess they think brown sugar isn't sugar.)
- 1/4 cup honey   (What *do* they think makes honey sweet? [16])
- 1 egg slightly beaten (1 egg yolk alone has 300 mg. of cholesterol)
- 5 tbs. melted butter   (Delicious but…die another day.)
- 1/2 c reduced fat milk (Only *reduced* fat?)

Nooooo! Bad! Are they trying to kill us?

So I've underlined the villains up there. Below is what I've replaced them with to make the **New Age Pancake:**

- 1/2 cup soy flour & 1/2 cup whole wheat pastry flour (to replace the all-purpose flour)
- 6 tablespoons Splenda (for the honey & brown sugar)
- 1 tablespoon baking powder
- 1/2 cup skim milk & 1/2 cup canola oil (to replace the "reduced" fat milk & melted butter)
- Egg Replacement, mix separately: 1 tbsp warm water; 1 heaping tbsp canola oil, 1 heaping tbsp baking powder. Three seconds & it'll start to fizz. Fun to watch. Then add to batter, and stir.

Spray large skillet with Pam &, on medium-high heat, drop some batter. If it looks too cakey, add more milk to batter. When bubbles appear, flip & cook other side. Serve hot. Makes 12 pancakes, **112 calories each.**

---

16   Maybe they think there's a special breed of bees that make honey with Splenda.

MLA Banana Oatmeal Muffins

Per Serving, 120 calories

Cooking spray
1 cup quick-cook oatmeal
1/2 cup whole wheat flour
1/2 cup Splenda
1 tablespoon double-acting baking powder
1/4 teaspoon ground ginger
1/2 teaspoon ground nutmeg
1 ripened banana
1/4 cup tofu, mashed
1/2 cup skim milk
3 tablespoons canola oil
1 tbsp Ener-G Egg Replacer + 1/4 cup warm water

Spray cooking spray on 9 three-inch muffin cups; preheat oven to 350. (Put small amount of water in any left over empty cups.)

1. Stir together oatmeal, wheat flour, Splenda, baking powder, ginger & nutmeg; set aside.
2. Mash tofu with banana; add in skim milk & canola oil.
3. Separately, mix egg replacer & warm water, then add to all other ingredients. Mix.
4. Pour into prepared muffin cups. Each cup should be about 2/3 full. Bake for 15 to 20 minutes, or until a tester comes out clean.
5. Cool on rack for 15 minutes

Makes 9 muffins, **120** calories each, Total carbs 9, Dietary carbs 2.2

(If walnuts added to mix & topping, 85 extra calories per muffin, or 205 calories each.)

Cheese & Veggies Pita Pocket

1 Joseph's Flax, oat bran & whole wheat pita (60 c.)
4 slices Fat Free cheese singles (30 c. each; 120 c. for four)
Dijon mustard
sliced tomato, lettuce, onion, fresh peppers, as desired

Cut small edge off pita, slice almost completely open like a book.
On a plate lightly spread on Dijon. Lay cheese singles on each side
of pita. Microwave for about 30 seconds or until cheese is soft.
Quickly lay on sliced vegetables (drained of excess water so pita
won't get soggy); then close the two pita sides.
Refrigerate for a few minutes so cheese will "set."

Per Serving: 200 calories, 20 g. protein, 8 g carbohydrates (of
which 4 Dietary Fiber), 2 g fat (0 saturated, 0 trans fat), 300
milligrams sodium, 20 milligrams cholesterol, calcium 60%
MDR

• • •

Tomato & cheese Pita

Joseph's pita, 1
Tomato, thickly sliced
fat-free cheese, 2 slices   30 calories each, 60 for 2

Place tomato slices between cheese slices, slip into pita,
microwave for 20 seconds or till cheese is gooey & will "glue"
tomato slices when pocket cools.
Optional: add olives or sliced red onions

125 calories per serving

Anytime Blondies™*

Grab 'n run – healthiest meal replacement: No sugar, No fat, 169 calories, & *19 g. protein* per serving. (A hamburger has 12 g protein; 4 oz nonfat yogurt 10 g; 8 oz of skim milk 8 grams; 1 egg white 5 grams.) Total Carbs,15 grams per Blondie, less than a slice of whole wheat bread.

Makes 9 big servings. Cut in half, these make filling snacks at **85** calories each.

Cooking spray
2 3/4 cups quick cook oatmeal...825 calories .... 27 grams protein
1 1/4 cup Splenda
*5 scoops Soy Protein Powder...275c .... 115 g protein
1/2 tsp salt
1 tbsp baking powder
2 tsp vanilla extract
1 tbsp canola ....20 c.
2 cups cold fat free milk + 1 oz pkg Jell-o sugar free <u>Vanilla</u> pudding .... 280 calories .... 19 g protein
1/4 cup fat free milk (in case batter too thick).........................22 .... 1 g protein

Preheat oven to 350. Ready two mixing bowls. Spray 8 x 8 inch bake dish.
In smaller bowl combine the oatmeal, Splenda, Protein Powder, salt, & baking powder.
In larger bowl, add vanilla & canola to milk, combine with Jello powder & whisk 2 minutes till pudding thickens. Add dry ingredients into pudding & mix well. Batter will be thick. Spread in pan & bake at 350 for 25-30 minutes. Better to cool before cutting.

*The star here is **Soy Protein Powder.** You can add more if you like. Each serving of 2 scoops (= 1/3 cup, 30 grams, or 1 ounce), has 110 calories and 23 grams of protein. It is fluffy, sweet, and can replace up to half the flour in many baking recipes. Try it too in Smoothies; sprinkle it in or on…anything. Pure protein, no fat, and nooo sugar.

Anytime Brownies™

Same* nutritional stats as Anytime Blondies except for more protein. Makes 9 servings, **185** calories & **21** grams protein each. Two differences here: 1) Unsweetened cocoa has been added because the Jello product is alkanized, or "Dutch processed," which destroys the antioxidants; and 2) two cups liquid egg whites have been substituted for the same amount of fat free milk. That adds even more protein. Total Carbs are the same as for Blondies.

*You can leave out the Soy Powder or cocoa if you feel you've enough protein or chocolate in your day's diet, making each serving considerably lower cal. (You won't need the extra 1/4 milk then, either.) Add more Splenda if you'd like the result sweeter.

Makes 9 servings. Cut in half: filling snacks at **93** calories each.

Cooking spray
2 3/4 cups quick cook oatmeal...................................825calories
.... 27 grams protein
1 1/2 cup Splenda
1/4 cup (4 tbsp) unsweetened cocoa ....80 c.
5 scoops Soy Protein Powder..275 c
.... 115 g protein
1/2 tsp salt
1 tbsp baking powder
1 tsp vanilla extract
1 tbsp canola ....120 c.
2 cups liquid egg whites..250 c.
.... 50 g protein
1 oz pkg just Jell-o sugar free <u>Chocolate </u>pudding .... 100 calories
1/4 cup fat free milk (if batter too thick)...............................22
.... 1 g protein

Preheat oven to 350. Ready two mixing bowls. Spray 8 x 8 inch bake dish.

In smaller bowl combine the oatmeal, Splenda, cocoa, Protein
Powder, salt, & baking powder.

In larger bowl, add vanilla & canola to egg whites, combine with
Jello powder & whisk 2 minutes. Add dry ingredients & mix well.
If batter's too thick add a bit more milk. Spread in pan & bake at
350 for 23-25 minutes. (The egg whites bake faster.) Cool before
cutting.

Anytime Cheese 'n Onions Bar™

Serves 9, 112 calories per serving.

Great grab & run meal, good for anytime. No bad flour & no sugar of any kind. Filling too, and more nutritious than most meals.

Cooking spray
1 1/2 cup quick cook oatmeal .... 450 calories
1/2 cup Splenda
1 tsp salt
1 tbsp baking powder
fresh ground pepper, to taste
large onion, sliced... 60 c.
sliced mushrooms .... 25 c.
garlic & more pepper, to taste
1 cup liquid egg whites .... 120 c.
2 cups fat free shredded cheddar cheese .... 360 c.

Preheat over to 350. In bowl combine the oatmeal, Splenda,salt & pepper to taste. Spray both skillet & 8" square cooking pan. Sautee onions & mushrooms, adding garlic & pepper. Lower heat. Pour eggs & cheese into skillet, stir until mixture's melted. Pour into bowl containing oatmeal mixture, stir well, then pour into greased pan. Bake at 350 for 25-30 minutes, or until inserted toothpick comes out clean. Let cool 5 minutes before cutting. Air dry further on cookie rack, if desired.

Anytime Cheese & Turkey Bar™

makes 9, 163 calories per serving.

Another great grab & run meal. Filling, full of fiber, protein, and more nutritious than most meals.

Cooking spray
1 1/2 cup quick cook oatmeal .... 450 calories
1/2 cup Splenda
1 tbsp baking powder
1 tsp salt
1 pound fat free ground turkey .... 480 calories
large onion, sliced... 60 c.
garlic & fresh ground pepper, to taste
1 cup cup liquid egg whites... 120 c.
2 cups fat free shredded cheddar cheese........................... 360 c.

Preheat over to 350. In large bowl combine the oatmeal, Splenda, baking powder & salt. Spray both skillet & 8" square cooking pan. Sautee onions & turkey, adding garlic & pepper to taste. Lower heat; pour off all drippings. Into skillet pour eggs & cheese, stir until cheese is melted. Pour all skillet contents into bowl containing oatmeal mixture, mix well, then pour into greased pan. Bake at 350 for 30 minutes, or until inserted toothpick comes out clean. Let cool 5 minutes before cutting. Air dry further on cookie rack, if desired.

Berry Intense Smoothie

Per serving, 75 calories

1/4 cup fat free sugar free yogurt
1 tsp artificial sweetener
1/4 cup raspberries, fresh or frozen
1/4 cup drained mandarin oranges
1/2 cup Diet Orange soda

Combine in a blender and mix until smooth.

Strawberry Smoothie .... 75 calories
1/2 cup fat-free milk... 40 c.
1/2 cup strawberries (frozen is ok)....................................... 50 c.
1/2 cup diet orange soda
6 tablespoons artificial sweetener

Combine yogurt, milk and artificial sweetener in blender. Add
berries & blend until smooth.

• • •

Chocolate Smoothies

Per Serving, 90 calories

1/2 cup non fat yogurt .... 50 calories
2 tbsp unsweetened cocoa .... 40 calories
2 tbsp Splenda or Equal
Diet Coke

In a measuring cup, mix first 3 ingredients well. Pour in a splash
of Diet Coke, mix, watch it froth. Add a bit more; mix until
smooth.
Pour whole mixture into tall glass, fill rest with Coke. Stick in a
straw.

Mocha Latte

1 cup heated fat-free milk.. 80 calories
1 tbsp unsweetened cocoa .... 20 calories
1 tbsp Splenda
2 tsp Instant Coffee (or Decaff)
1/8 teaspoon ground cinnamon (optional)

Place milk, cocoa, Splenda, coffee and cinnamon in blender. Cover
& blend until smooth.

100 calories per serving

Rye & Cheese Sandwich Per serving: .... 270 calories

2 slices rye bread with sesame seeds .... 180 calories
1 tbsp Dijon
3 slices Fat Free Cheese Singles... 90 c.
tomato slices

Make sandwich, tomato slices alternating with the cheese.
Microwave about 20 seconds

Scrambled eggs & cheese pita: Per serving, ... 135 calories

Cooking spray
1 pita (Joseph's Oat Bran & Whole Wheat pita if possible).. 60c.
1/4 cup liquid egg whites... 30 calories
1/4 cup shredded fat-free cheese............................... 45 calories
garlic & pepper to taste
Dijon mustard if desired.

Coat frying pan with cooking spray. Spread Dijon inside the pita,
if desired.

Whisk eggs and cheese, then cook egg mixture, garlic & pepper
on low-medium heat, until cheese is melted & egg looks done.
Quickly spoon scrambled egg mixture into pita before cheese
cools.

MLA Mini-quiches

freezes well; also good for lunch, snacks. Recipe below makes 4.

No-Stick Cooking Spray
1/2 cup liquid egg whites .... 64 c
1/2 cup fat free shredded cheddar cheese .... 90 c
1/4 cup sliced onions
1/4 cup sliced mushrooms
dried garlic, cinnamon & nutmeg to taste

Preheat oven to 350 degrees. Spray paper/foil cups with cooking
spray. Arrange in muffin pans.
Coat skillet with cooking spray. Sautee onions and mushrooms,
add spices & lower heat. Add liquid eggs, cheese & stir till cheese
melts. Mixture will be beigey "mush." Don't worry. Divide evenly
into muffin cups, filling each 2/3 full
Bake at 350 for 15-17 minutes, or until toothpick inserted in
center comes out clean. Let cool before storing in freezer

Per Serving: 45 calories per quiche

• • •

Turkey rollups

Per serving: 215 calorie

1 Joseph's Oat Bran & Whole Wheat tortilla
1 slice of deli turkey
3 pieces fat free singles cheese
2 teaspoons Dijon mustard
3 medium lettuce leaves

Place tortilla on plate & spread Dijon. Place 2 cheese pieces
lengthwise; break 3rd piece in half & put on empty sides.
Microwave (still on plate) until cheese is soft. Quickly lay on
lettuce & turkey slice; roll up with fold side down. Place in fridge
for a few minutes, even freezer for quick chill

Tuna Melt Rollup

Per serving, 255 calories

1 Joseph's Oat Bran & Whole Wheat tortilla
3 slices fat free cheese
2oz Solid White Albacore Tuna (in water)
chopped onions
1/4 cup Mayonnaise Healthy Substitute

To the mayonnaise substitute add tuna & onion, mix all. Place
tortilla on a plate, arrange cheese slices on it, microwave tortilla
& cheese about 35-40 seconds. Remove; quickly spread line of
tuna mix across the circle, stopping 2" from the edges. Roll up,
starting at the shorter side. Tuck in ends like a business envelope;
lay rollups to cool seam side down.

• • •

Crunchy Fruit rollup

Per serving, 250 calories

1 Joseph's pita
3 slices fat free cheese
5 walnut halves, broken into chunks
1/2 cup seedless red grapes, sliced in half (to roll up more easily).

Cut pita & place open like a book on plate. Arrange 2 cheese
slices; tear 3rd piece in half to fit empty spaces. Microwave cheese-
covered pita 45 seconds. Remove, sprinkle walnuts & grapes, roll
up & place with fold side down.

Entrees

MLA Chicken Marsala,

serves 4…double or triple recipe using 2 or 3 skillets; use for lunch 1 or 2 days later; freeze leftovers

1 pound skinless, boneless, chicken breasts, trimmed of fat
1 tbsp bottled minced garlic
1 teaspoon dried tarragon (or more)
8 oz sliced mushrooms
1/4 cup dry marsala
1/2 cup fat free, no sodium chicken broth
optional: 1 tbsp Splenda
sprinkled black pepper

Spray pan with cooking spray. Lay chicken breasts on plate & lightly sprinkle with pepper. Over medium high heat sauté chicken 3-4 minutes on each side until lightly browned. Remove chicken to plate.
Add garlic, tarragon, and mushrooms; sauté until mushrooms turn golden.
Add wine, cook 1 minute. Stir in broth. Add Splenda if mixture needs sweetening.
Return chicken to pans. Cover with wine mixture, simmer for 2 to 3 minutes until equally heated and slightly thickened.
Place 4 ounces of chicken on each of 4 plates, topping each with the marsala and mushroom sauce.

Per Serving: 250 calories, 25 g protein, 7 g fat (0 trans fat; 10 g monounsaturated, 1.5 polyunsaturated, 2 saturated), 25 mg cholesterol, sodium 55 mg.

MLA Tex Mex chicken

(Make a ton of this. It's one of the most nutrient-packed of all recipes & freezes well. Divide into 1-lb Ziplocs, freezer or lunch containers)

Serves 4

Cooking spray
3 pounds chicken tenderloins
Frozen broccoli florets, whole bag or nearly
Frozen, shelled soy beans, or Edamame
2-3 yellow squash, pre-cut, best stored in Ziploc with peppers, below
Peppers, red & orange, cut into pretty strips & squares (can be cut & frozen ahead. Store-bought are less pretty. Too shreddy-looking)
1 bottle low sugar barbecue sauce

Spray Skillet with cooking spray. Cut chicken into small chunks. Over medium high heat, sautee chicken until golden. Pour off all drippings, leave chicken in pan. Add whole bottle of barbecue sauce, frozen broccoli, yellow squash, red & orange peppers. Reheat all, stirring occasionally, adding more water if sauce too thick
Let simmer and serve in 4 oz portions

Per Serving: 215 calories

Fettucini Alfredo

*Tofu Shirataki Fettuccini Noodles..............................20 calories
1/4 cup (62 g) of 15 oz Fat Free Ricotta cheese ....50 c.
1/2 c. skim milk ....40 c.
1 tbsp olive oil..120
3 slices Fat Free White Singles Cheese, torn into pieces ... 90 cal.
3 tbsp garlic, powdered
pepper to taste

Mix together ricotta & skim milk; set aside. Rinse noodles well & microwave for one minute.
Add olive oil, stir. Then add white cheese, let melt & fold in.
Add milk-ricotta mixture, garlic, & pepper to taste; mix.
Serve hot. If desired, top with shrimp or sliced, baked chicken.

Fettuccin per serving: **320** calories, Total carbs 9, Dietary carbs 2

- Dreamfields as of this writing doesn't yet make Fettucini. You could substitute their linguini at 190 calories per 2 oz serving.
- Dreamfields has 1/8 the carbs of regular pizza, & some believe it tastes better. On the other hand Shirataki Fettuccini, at 1/30 the carbs & **20** calories per serving, is a filling & super fast way to lose weight.

Salmon Dijon

Cooking spray
Heavy duty aluminum foil
4 oz salmon
1 teaspoon Dijon mustard (5 cal. per person)
Garlic powder
Dill, dried

Figure 4 oz salmon per person. Buy as much as you'll need, and cut into 4 oz pieces

Line broiling platter with aluminum foil & spray with cooking spray.
Place salmon fillets on foil
"Finger paint" Dijon over each fillet
Balance platter over sink; sprinkle on lots of garlic powder and dill
Broil (2nd shelf down) until Dijon topping starts to brown
Close oven door & switch to bake for another 2-3 minutes, or until fillets are browned and easily "flaked." Dijon mixture prevents them from drying
Let cool slightly. Peel away skins & serve.

salmon (4 ounces): 230 calories

Per serving: 265 calories, 13 g fat, 0 g carbs, 20 g protein

Crudites

(pronounced crudi*tay*; means any raw veggies appetizer or side dish)

1/4 cup Broccoli florets, raw & cut small
1/4 cup Carrots, cut small
1/4 cup Tomatoes, diced
per serving: 75 calories
Arrange on plate or side dish, drizzle with Vinaigrette

• • •

*MLA Vinaigrette

...Indispensable, used in many recipes. Make lots & keep handy in fridge. Suggested container: old Dijon jar.

Serves 4:
4 tablespoons extra virgin olive oil
2 tablespoons red wine vinegar
2 teaspoons Dijon mustard
garlic powder
tarragon, dried

Pour olive oil into container. Add red wine vinegar, then Dijon; stir.
Add powdered garlic & tarragon. Lots.
Stir with fork, or if using old Dijon jar, screw cover back on and shake vigorously.
Recipe thus far is your true vinaigrette. If you wish fewer calories in it add more water, screw cover back on, and shake again. You can add more garlic & tarragon; the calorie count won't change & they're what really gives vinaigrette its taste.

125 calories per serving

MLA Western Omelet, Per serving: 215 calories

Cooking spray
1/2 cup onion, sliced.. 30 calories
1/2 cup mushrooms, sliced .... 10 calories
1/2 cup sun-dried tomatoes .... 70 calories
1/2 cup liquid egg whites... 60 calories
1/4 cup shredded fat-free cheese.............................. 45 calories

Coat frying pan with cooking spray. Sautee onions and mushrooms, add tomatoes last, sautee another minute. Toss in egg whites and cheese, cook & stir till done, serve hot.

• • •

MLA Lemon-Garlic Marinated Shrimp

Cooking spray
2 tablespoons minced garlic
10 med. cooked *shrimp .... 55 calories
1 cup cherry tomatoes, sliced............................... 30 c.
1/4 cup lemon juice
1/4 cup fresh parsley
salt & pepper to taste

Spray pan with cooking spray. Sautee garlic in over medium heat until golden, about 1 minute. Add tomatoes & shrimp; cook for an additional two minutes. Add 1/4 cup lemon juice, 1/4 cup minced parsley and salt and pepper to taste.
Toss all together, remove from heat

Per serving: 100 calories

*About 5.5 calories per shrimp

Stir Fry Vegetables

Cooking spray
1/2 cup broccoli florets
1/2 cup sliced carrots
1 sliced onion
3/4 cup chicken broth
1 tablespoon cornstarch
1/4 cup cold water
1 small can sliced water chestnuts, drained
1/2 cup sliced mushrooms
1/2 cup sugar peas

Spray skillet with cooking oil and heat until hot
Add broccoli, carrots and onion; stir-fry 1 minute
Lower heat. Add chicken broth and cook until carrots are crisp-tender, about 2 minutes
Mix cornstarch into cold water; add to vegetables and stir until thickened, about 20 seconds
Add water chestnuts, sugar peas, and mushrooms last. Cook & stir 30 seconds more

Per Serving: 225 calories

Tuna Vinaigrette

Serves 2

1/2 cup Vinaigrette
1/2 bag frozen broccoli florets
1/2 cup frozen shelled soybeans (Edamame)
1 6 oz can of tuna
1 can (15 oz) red or dark kidney beans, drained
1 can sliced small black olives
small onion, sliced
2 small tomatoes, diced

Pour the vinaigrette into skillet. Add broccoli and Edamame, heating till thawed. Add water to stretch sauce further with fewer calories. Lower heat, add tuna, kidney beans, & olives, stirring until evenly warmed.
Add tomatoes & onions last, stir briefly but leave onions crunchy

320 calories per person

MLA Chicken Cacciatore

serves 4, nutrient-intense, double or triple recipe using 2 or 3 skillets; use for lunch & freeze leftovers

Cooking Spray
1 pound chicken breasts
4 tablespoons bottled minced garlic
8 oz sliced mushrooms
1/2 bag frozen broccoli florets
1/2 bag frozen spinach
1 can pasta paste
1/2 cup of water
2 tbsp olive oil
1 cup fat free, no sodium chicken broth
2 teaspoons dried basil
2 teaspoons dried oregano
1/2 teaspoon black pepper
1 lg. sliced onion

Spray skillet with cooking spray and cut chicken into small pieces. Over medium high heat sautee garlic, mushrooms, and chicken until golden.
Pour off any drippings.
Lower heat & push chicken mixture to one side.
In cleared place add whole can of pasta paste. Slowly stir in the water, olive oil, chicken broth, basil, pepper, oregano, & more powdered garlic if desired.
Stir & mix sauce. Add broccoli florets and spinach. Simmer whole mixture, stirring in onions last so they'll be crunchy.

Per serving: 245 calories

MLA Chicken Tarragon

with grapes & walnuts (grapes freeze well)

4 skinless, boneless, chicken breasts, trimmed of fat
black pepper
3 tbsp powdered garlic
3 tbsp dried tarragon
1/2 cup Vinaigrette
1/2 cup walnuts, broken into chunky pieces
1 cup red seedless grapes, cut in half lengthwise

Spray skillet with cooking spray. Place chicken breasts on plate & sprinkle with pepper. On medium high heat sauté on each side until lightly browned, adding garlic and tarragon. Lower heat, pour in vinaigrette. Stir, gently mixing in pan scrapings. Add walnuts & grapes last. Simmer for 2 to 3 minutes, then top chicken breasts with the vinaigrette/grapes/walnuts sauce.

Serves 4
Per Serving: **255** calories

This also makes a terrific salad, cut up and tossed with lettuce.

Linguine with White Clam Sauce

serves 2

4 oz Dreamfields Linguini (1/8th the carbs of regular pasta)
2 cans minced clams
1 tbsp olive oil
fresh cut or dried parsley
1 tbsp garlic, powdered

In saucepan cook clams & their juice on medium-high heat for five minutes. Add olive oil, garlic, & parsley.

Prepare linguini according to package directions. Drain. Arrange minced clam & broth over linguini; serve hot.

Per serving, 335 calories

• • •

Nova Scotia omelet

Cooking spray
3 oz Nova Scotia salmon ....115 c.
1/2 cup liquid egg whites ....60 c.
1/4 cup mushrooms
1 small onion, sliced into wide transverse sections

Spray skillet with cooking spray. On high heat, sautee mushrooms & onions (Carmelize wide onion slices on one side, then the other, turning carefully. They should look brown-glazed and artistic.)
Move still-browning onions to one side, lower heat slightly, and pour in eggs & salmon. Stir, mixing in with the mushrooms. Or, you can place pieces of salmon atop the mushrooms here & there, like a pizza. Garnish with the caramelized onions.

225 calories per serving

Spaghetti & *MLA meatballs

per serving **250** calories, including sauce & pasta (Make tons of meatballs!) Recipe below serves 5.

Meatballs:
1 20 oz (1.25 lbs) pkg of 99 % Fat-Free Ground Turkey
1 can tomato paste
1 medium onion, diced
3 tablespoons garlic, powdered
1 1/2 tablespoons dried oregano
1 1/2 tablespoons dried basil

Line a broiler pan with heavy foil. Spray foil with cooking spray and set aside. In a large bowl, combine the turkey, tomato paste, onion, egg whites, & spices. Shape "meatballs" & arrange on sprayed pan. About 3 should equal a 4 oz serving
Broil until tops are slightly brown and then turn and broil the other sides.
Set turkey balls to drain on Bounty-covered plate.

Meat balls per 4 oz serving: **160** calories, 1 g fat, 70 mg cholesterol, 55 mg sodium, 0 g carbohydrate, 28 g protein

Tomato Sauce:
1 can tomato paste
1 1/2 tbsp extra virgin olive oil
dried garlic, oregano, & basil, adjusted to taste
1 1/2 cup water
Combine all above slowly in skillet, stirring. **70** calories per 1/2 cup

Shirataki Noodles: **20** calories per 4 oz serving. (Really.) Follow directions on pkge. (Shirataki: 1/30th the carbs. Dreamfields noodles taste better but have 1/8th the carbs & 190 calories per 2 oz. Serving.)

Garlic Shrimp & Vegetables

Cooking spray
1 tablespoon minced garlic
1/4 cup broccoli florets
1/4 cup diagonally sliced carrots
1 small onion, sliced & separated into rings
1/2 cup chicken broth
1 tablespoon cornstarch
1/4 cup cold water
1/2 can (4 oz) drained, sliced water chestnuts
1/4 cup sliced mushrooms
1/4 cup sugar snap peas
1 teaspoons dried ginger
1/2 cup shelled, cooked shrimp, medium size

Spray skillet with cooking spray and heat until hot.
Add garlic, stir-fry until light brown.
Add broccoli, carrots and onion, stir-fry 1 minute
Add chicken broth, simmer for about 2 minutes
Mix cornstarch & cold water; stir into vegetable mixture. Continue stirring until thickened, about 15 seconds.
Add water chestnuts, mushrooms, and shrimp; cook and stir 30 seconds more

Per serving: 275 calories

Polynesian Chicken

Serves 2, Per serving: 245 calories

Preheat oven to 350

Heavy duty aluminum foil
2 chicken breasts
4 Tbsp Sweet & Sour Sauce
1/4 cup canned mandarin oranges, drained
1/4 cup canned pineapple chunks, drained

Line broiling platter with aluminum foil & spray with cooking spray.
Cover chicken breasts on both sides with sauce, & place on foil
Bake at 350 degrees for 25 minutes
Remove from oven. Turn breasts over, sprinkle the orange & pineapple chunks, baste all with the sauce
Return to oven. Bake for another 20 minutes, or until breasts and fruit start to brown

MLA Chili

For an any-time crowd pleaser. Make it by the truckload.

Cooking spray
3 skillets
3 20 oz (1.25 lbs) pkgs 99 % Fat-Free GroundTurkey
2 28 oz cans Crushed Tomatoes
3 medium onions, diced
Taco Seasoning Mix, 2 packets per pound of turkey
3 cans Dark Kidney Beans

Spray each skillet with cooking spray. Sautee the turkey throroughly. (More effort is required stirring/separating ground-turkey "crumbles" than with high-fat, slippery ground beef.)
Lower heat. Pour off all drippings. Add the crushed tomatoes, onions, and Taco Seasoning. Stir.
Add kidney beans, stir again, and let simmer for 5 minutes.

Per 4 oz serving: 210 calories

Serve with diced tomatoes, shredded lettuce, & fat-free cheese if desired. For that add 30 calories for each cheese slice.

MLA Chicken Stroganoff

(healthy variation on beef stronganoff)

4 boneless, skinless chicken breast halves
ground pepper to taste
1 medium onion, chopped
1/2 pound fresh mushrooms, sliced
3/4 cup chicken broth
2 tbsp garlic, dried
2 tbsp tarragon, dried
1/2 container Fat Free Sour Cream (8 oz)

Spray skillet with cooking spray. Rinse chicken breasts, trim fat, cut into smaller pieces, & sprinkle with pepper.
Over medium-high heat, cook chicken until golden on one side. Turn, sautee other side. Push pieces to far side of skillet & pour off any drippings.
Add onion ; cook until softened. Add garlic, tarragon, & mushrooms; cook for 2 more minutes.
Stir in chicken broth, stir, & lower heat.
Add sour cream, & stir chicken into rest of mixture. Cover chicken with sauce & simmer for 5 minutes, stirring occasionally.

Makes 4 servings, **235** calories each

Serve over cooked noodles, if desired. (Dreamfield's or Shirataki)

Dreamfield's, 1/8th the carbs of regular pasta. Serving size: 2 oz (they swell), **190** calories, Total Fat 1 g, 0 g saturated fat, 0 mg cholesterol, 0 g sugar, total carbs 42 g (dietary carbs, 5 g)

Tofu Shirataki Noodles: 1/30th the carbs of regular pasta. Serving size 2 oz, **20** calories. Each liquid-filled, chilled, package contains 2 servings.
Total fat 0.5 g, saturated fat 0 g, cholesterol 0 mg, Sugar 0 g, Total carbs 3 g

*MLA Lasagna

(Use Dreamfields: 65% lower glycemic index than regular pasta, only 5 g digestible carbs, 95 calories per 10x3"noodle. Available at DreamfieldsFoods.com & Amazon.com if not locally)

9 pieces Dreamfields Lasagna
2 lbs Fat Free Ground Turkey
1 medium onion, diced
3 tablespoons powdered garlic
1 1/2 dried oregano
1 1/2 tbsp dried basil
1/2 tbsp nutmeg
1 container (15 oz) Fat Free Ricotta cheese
1 pkg Fat Free Mozzarella cheese, shredded
3 cups tomato sauce

In large bowl, combine turkey, onion, & spices. Set aside.
Prepare lasagna according to package directions. Drain & rinse in cool water.
In large skillet, on medium heat, brown turkey mixture, stirring, until no long pink. Drain all juices. Preheat over to 375. Spray a 13x9x3 baking dish with Pam. Mix ricotta & mozzarella together.
Spread thin layer tomato sauce over bottom of 9"x13" baking dish. Layer 3 lasagna pieces side by side. Spread with 1/3 cheese mixture, 1/2 the turkey, & more tomato sauce.
Layer 3 more lasagna pieces, 1/3 cheese mixture, & more tomato sauce. Layer 3 more lasagna pieces, remaining cheese, turkey mixture, & tomato sauce.
Bake for 25 minutes. Remove and bake 10 more minutes. Let stand 10 minutes before cutting.

Serves 8.
325 calories per serving

MLA Shrimp Scampi

Cooking spray
1 lb pre-cooked shrimp
black pepper to taste
1 tbsp minced garlic
1 tbsp freshly chopped parsley
1 tbsp freshly squeezed lemon juice

Season shrimp with pepper. Spray skillet with cooking spray. Add
shrimp & garlic to skillet on high heat & stir for 2 minutes
Lower heat to medium, add lemon juice. Stir, scraping in any
browned bits from bottom of pan for 45 seconds.
Add parsley to sauce, toss to combine.

Number of Servings: 4,   215 calories per serving

MLA Chicken Parmigiana

Cooking spray
Four boneless, skinless chicken breasts
12 oz can tomato paste
1 tbsp olive oil
1 1/2 cup water
dried garlic, oregano, & basil, to taste
4 slices Fat Free Cheese

Spray wide skillet with cooking spray.
On medium-high heat, sear chicken breasts on both sides. Lower heat. Continue to cook chicken until nearly done. Pour off all drippings.
Push cooked breasts to one side. Into same pan push the tomato paste.
Stirring, add the water, olive oil and spices. If sauce too thick add more water.
Move the cooked breasts back into the sauce. Mix, cover breasts, let simmer a few minutes. Cover each breast with one slice of Fat Free cheese. Let melt for about 2 minutes. Transfer cheese-covered chicken & sauce to plates, and serve

4 servings, 253 calories each

Penne Rigate with Chicken, Mushrooms, & Broccoli

Serves 4

Cooking spray
8 oz Penne Rigate (Dreamfields recommended: 1/8 the carbs of regular pasta. As of this writing Shirataki Tofu noodles, with 1/30 the carbs of regular pasta, don't yet manufacture Penne)
1/2 cup chopped onion
1/2 cup sliced fresh mushrooms
3 boneless, skinless chicken breasts, cut into smaller pieces
2 tbsp garlic, powdered
pepper to taste
1 cup broccoli florets (fresh or frozen)
extra virgin olive oil, 1 tbsp.
6 No Fat cheese slices

Spray large skillet with cooking spray. Over medium heat sauté onion & mushrooms till both turn golden.
Add chicken, garlic, & pepper; cook 10 minutes or until meat is no longer pink. Add broccoli, cook for another 3 minutes.
Meanwhile, cook pasta according to package directions. Drain, add olive oil, 4 cheese slices, & melt into pasta
Combine chicken mixture to pasta; toss. Top with remaining cheese slices torn into pieces. Brown under broiler for 3-5 minutes, and serve.

per serving: **340** calories

Desserts and Healthy Sweets

Fudge Sauce

Mix together equal amounts of Unsweetened (non-alkalinized) Cocoa & Splenda. Add water a bit at a time, stirring, till sauce reaches desired consistency. Microwave if you like, pour on yogurt, fruit, anything. Each tbsp unsweetened cocoa = 20 calories. **Two tablespoons** mixed with water make a nice serving: **40 calories.** No sugar, no fat --

-- and a mega-dose of antioxidants. **One tablespoon = 15 grams.** Figure there are 7 tablespoons per 100 grams, & look at the list below:

Top 10 Antioxidant Foods According to USDA Research
(per 100 grams)
1. Unsweetened Cocoa Powder ....26,000 ORACs*
2. Dark Chocolate...13,120
3. Blueberries 2,400
4. Strawberries..1,540
5. Spinach...1,260
6. Raspberries...1,220
7. Red Grapes..739

*Means **Oxygen Radical Absorbance Capacity**, a fancy way of measuring how well a certain food will help your body fight diseases like cancer and heart disease." The higher the number, the better.
*For unsweetened cocoa, 26,000 per 100 grams = 260 per gram. Two tbsp = 30 grams, so it's 30 x 260 = 7,800 ORACs in 2 tablespoons unsweetened cocoa, <u>3,900 ORACs per tablespoon</u>. That's amazing. Hyper-boosts your health.

Chocolate Berry Parfait

1/4 banana, sliced
3 sliced strawberries
1/4 cup blueberries
2 tbsp fudge sauce
4 oz non-fat, sugar-free yogurt
1 tsp artificial sweetener
1 tsp Jello Orange, Lime, Black Cherry etc. flavor

Arrange fruits in dessert cup(s). Heat fruit mixture 40 seconds in microwave. (Creates sophisticated-looking pool of berry juice.) Stir artificial sweetener into the yogurt; spoon yogurt onto fruits; top all with fudge sauce.

Per Serving: **120** calories

• • •

Orange Walnut Mousse with Fudge Sauce

4 oz non-fat sugar-free yogurt
1 tsp artificial sweetener
1 tsp Sugar-free Orange Jello
2 walnut halves, chopped
2 tbsp fudge sauce

Chop walnuts
Stir artificial sweetener, Sugar-free Orange Jello, & walnuts into yogurt
Spoon into dessert cups
Top with fudge sauce

Per serving , **120** calories

Fudge Nut Tart

*To make chocolate candies, keep fillo plastic trays.

15 Athens Mini Fillo Shells (1 box), each shell 18 calories
1/2 cup (8 tbsp) unsweetened cocoa .... 160 calories
1/2 cup Splenda
10 walnut halves... 100 calories

Mix equal parts unsweetened cocoa & Splenda. Add cold water, just enough to make fudgey mixture thick. Add chopped walnuts, stir. Using soup spoon, transfer into two small plastic bags, pushing mixture toward one of the doubled bags' corners. Twist like a pastry bag & snip tiny piece off bags' corner. Hold fillo tarts one at a time & squeeze bag, pushing fudge mixture into tart. Rotate as you squeeze, lifting bag up and away when nearly done.

15 tarts, each **35** calories & super healthy with antioxidants & omega-3 from the walnuts.

• • •

Pear, Pudding & Chocolate Sauce

2 pear halves, drained
Jello Sugar-Free Fat-Free Instant Lemon Pudding
2 cups cold, fat free milk
1 tbsp chocolate sauce
Fat Free whipped topping

Add Vanilla Pudding mix to milk. Whisk for two minutes, til mixture thickens. Pour into dessert cups. Then place 1 pear half on 1/2 cup of pudding, **80** calories. Top with Chocolate Sauce, **20** calories, and Fat Free whipped topping if desired, **15** calories per 2 tbsp serving.

Per serving: 115 calories

Apple Crisp with Whipped Topping

4 medium sliced tart apples
1/4 cup Whole Wheat Pastry Flour
1/4 cup Soy Flour
1 jar Sugar Free Apricot Preserves
1/4 cup Splenda
2 Minute Maid 'Just 10' Fruit punch
3/4 teaspoon ground cinnamon
3/4 teaspoon ground nutmeg

Peel & slice apples, some pieces in irregular chunks; set aside.
Preheat oven to 375. Spray cooking spray on 8x8 pan.

On medium heat in dry pan, "toast" the soy flour till it browns slightly.
Lower heat, melt Sugar Free Apricot Preserves into the soy. (If "mush" starts to stick to pan, remove from heat, stir bottom, then return to heat.)
Add both 'Just 10' Fruit Punch & Splenda; stir.
Add cinnamon, nutmeg, & Whole Wheat Pastry Flour. Combine well.
Press into baking dish to form a thin crust.
Arrange apples over the crust.

Bake about 30 minutes, or until top is golden and apples are tender.
Serve with Fat Free whipped topping & Chocolate Sauce if desired.

Serves 6.
Per serving: 103 calories.
With Fat Free whipped topping, 118 calories
With whipped topping & 1 tbsp Fudge Sauce, 138 calories

Chocolate Ice Cream with Whipped Topping

(Or **Vanilla** Ice Cream, **Lemon, Banana, White Chocolate,** & other flavors using Jello Sugar-Free Fat-Free Instant Puddings. Same calories, sweetened with safe Aspartame.)

1 pkg Jello Sugar-Free Fat-Free Instant Chocolate Fudge Pudding
2 cups cold Fat Free milk optional: Fat-Free whipped topping, fudge sauce, strawberries, etc.

Follow package directions to make pudding. Freeze in bowl for 1 1/2 hours. Take out, quickly re-stir to aereate, return to freezer for another 1/2 hour. (The trick is in the aeration. Ice cream machines churn constantly. If Ben & Jerry's were to use the best ingredients without this aeration, the result would be tasty ice.)

The ice cream alone is **70** calories per 1/2 cup serving.
Fat Free Whipped Topping is **15** calories per 2 tablespoons
2 tbsp fudge sauce (p. 109) added to those is another **40** calories, or **125** calories for all three.
If you don't freeze the pudding…it's pudding! Vanilla is luscious with fudge sauce & whipped topping, and the same 125 calories

• • •

Fruit Chocolate Fondue

5 strawberries, halved
1/2 apple, sliced thin with skin left on (anti-oxidants are on the dark-pigmented skin)
melon slices, whatever's in season
2 tbsp fudge sauce

Line outside rim of dessert dish with pretty fruits. In smaller dish or cup microwave fudge sauce for 20 seconds. Remove, place in center of fruits on larger dessert dish. Fork fruits & dip into warm chocolate.

Per Serving: 140 calories

Chocolate pudding with strawberries & topping

Jello Sugar-Free Fat-Free Instant Chocolate pudding
2 tbsp unsweetened *cocoa
2 tbsp Splenda
2 cups cold fat free milk
1/2 cup sliced strawberries

Serves 4, 93 calories per serving

Combine pudding mix with cocoa & Splenda. Stir in milk & whisk for 2-3 minutes until pudding thickens. Pour into dessert cups & arrange sliced strawberries on top.

*Add unsweetened cocoa because the Jello product is alkanized, or "Dutch processed," which destroys the antioxidants.

• • •

Diet Cappuccino

Make your regular coffee, pour into mugs or cups & add artificial sweetener if desired. In a fridge container, keep a small amount of lactose fat free *milk; maybe 4" inches at the bottom. Shake it vigorously; it will foam up fast. Pour the milky froth onto your coffee like a topping. Then sprinkle with <u>cinnamon</u>. Pretty. No calories. And cinnamon's full of antioxidants.

*Helps if the milk has been standing at room temp for about 20 minutes.

*Sprinkle with Cocoa too, if desired: 1 tsp Unsweetened Cocoa mixed with 1 tsp artificial sweetener.

Chocolate Mousse

Pkge Jell-O Sugar-Free Fat-Free Chocolate Pudding (serves 4)
4 tbsp unsweetened cocoa*
4 tbsp Splenda
2 tbsp whole grain oat flour (18 calories each tbsp)
1 3/4 cups cold fat-free milk
1/2 cup *room-temperature* egg whites
1/2 tsp cream of tartar

Preheat oven to 350 degrees.

In one bowl, mix together dry pudding mix, the unsweetened cocoa, Splenda, and oat flour. Add the milk and whisk 2-3 minutes until pudding mixture thickens.

In another bowl, beat egg whites till they start to become foamy. Add the cream of tartar, continue beating until whites "peak."

Fold together egg whites and pudding, pour mousse into 4 individual cups, and bake for 13 minutes.

100 calories per serving!

*Natural unsweetened cocoa is added because the pudding product contains alkanized cocoa.

New Age Brownies

More delicate than Anytime Brownies, and a very different kind of recipe. Still no bad fat, egg yolks -- or sugar in the form of mashed bananas, dates, honey, molasses & its other disguises. (You get plenty of sugar from the healthy grains, fruits, & veggies you eat. Metabolism's bottom line: EVERYTHING breaks down to one of three things: protein, fat, or sugar.)

Quick cook oatmeal, 1/2 cup .... 150 calories
Oat flour, 3/4 cup .... 225 c.
1 tablespoon baking powder
1 tsp salt
3/4 cup Unsweetened Cocoa .... 240 c.
1 cup Splenda
1 tbsp Ener-G egg replacer & 6 tbsp warm water
1 tsp vanilla extract
1 cup liquid egg whites .... 250 c.
*1/2 cup shredded fat free mozzarella cheese...................... 90 c.
5 tbsp canola oil .... 600 c.

Preheat oven to 350. Spray baking dish with cooking spray.
Mix 6 dry ingredients in medium bowl; set aside.
Separately fork-froth the Ener-G & water, then add vanilla.
Combine egg whites, cheese, & canola. Cook in skillet over low-medium heat, stirring as the cheese melts, adding the Ener-G mixture & vanilla. If eggs start to cook, remove from heat for a bit, stir more. Now add dry ingredients to mixture in pan, stir, pour into baking dish.
Bake for 15 minutes. Let cool 10-15 minutes before cutting.

Makes 16 snack-sized brownies, 97 calories each, or 12 huge brownies, 130 calories each. In each 12-size brownie: 5 g protein, 2 g dietary carbs.

* The cheese is what binds, like sugar & egg yolks.
* For fudgey topping, frost unbaked batter with thin layer of this diet's chocolate sauce.

Luscious Healthy Frosting

Enough for 6-7 muffins or cupcakes, 18 calories each.

4 oz plain non-fat or Greek yogurt............................ 50 calories
1 packet of artificial sweetener
1 level tsp Jello Sugar Free Fat Free Instant Pudding or Gelatin
(any flavor).. 20 c.
1 tsp canola oil .... 40 c.

Mix all ingredients together. 110 calories per 1/2 cup. Recommended
flavors: <u>Orange</u>, <u>Lime</u>, <u>Black Cherry</u>, <u>Vanilla</u>, <u>Lemon</u>,**<u>Chocolate</u>

For a richer, darker **Fudge Frosting:
2 tablespoons unsweetened cocoa....................................... 40 c.
2 tablespoons Splenda
1-2 tbsp water
1/2 teaspoon canola.. 20 c.

Mix all together. This will frost about two cupcakes or muffins,
at **30** calories per serving. It's more calories, but still, no sugar,
no butter, nothing bad -- and a mega-dose of antioxidants. **One
tablespoon = 15 grams.** Figure there are 7 tablespoons in 100
grams, & look at the list below:

Top 10 Antioxidant Foods According to USDA Research
(per 100 grams)
1. Unsweetened Cocoa Powder ....26,000 ORACs*
2. Dark Chocolate..13,120
3. Blueberries 2,400
4. Strawberries..1,540
5. Spinach...1,260
6. Raspberries..1,220
7. Red Grapes..739

*Means **Oxygen Radical Absorbance Capacity**, a fancy way of
measuring how well a certain food will help your body fight diseases

like cancer and heart disease." The higher the number, the better. ***For Fudge Frosting (unsweetened cocoa), 26,000 per 100 grams = 260 per gram. Two tbsp = 30 grams, so it's 30 x 260 = 7,800 ORACs in 2 tablespoons unsweetened cocoa.** That's amazing. Tops for your health.

● ● ●

Chocolate Candy

about 10 calories each if that much.

Natural Unsweetened Cocoa.........................20 calories per tbsp
Equal amount Splenda as Cocoa
Water
Optional, *walnuts................. (200 calories per 1/4 cup ground)
Plastic molds: Athens Mini Fillo Shell Molds or candy molds.

Mix Unsweetened Cocoa, Splenda, & water till mixture is thick & fudgey. Add ground nuts if desired. Spoon mixture into two small plastic Baggies or Ziplocs, push toward one corner of bags, twisting top like a pastry bag. With scissors cut off small tip of one corner, & squeeze fudge into plastic "discs" of original fillo tray or other plastic candy molds. Let air dry, then pop out. No need for cooking spray, just pop 'em out.

*Tip: When all molds are filled, raise mold tray & drop hard onto counter. Repeat if necessary. (Chocolate makers' trick: makes goo spread & gets the bubbles out.)

Air dry overnight, or, faster: freeze for 20-30 minutes (they'll still re-soften since they contain no fat & sugar to make them solid at room temperature).

*<u>Walnuts</u> are a top source of omega-3 acids to improve your cardiovascular health.

Black Cherry Chocolate Mousse

3 walnut halves
4 banana slices
2 sliced fresh or frozen strawberries
4 oz non-fat sugar-free yogurt
1 teaspoon Sugar-free Black Cherry Jello
Unsweetened Cocoa & artificial sweetener, 2 tbsp each.

Chop walnuts. Line dessert cups with fruit pieces; microwave 40 seconds.
Stir the sweetener, Sugar-free Black Cherry Jello, & walnuts into yogurt. Pour onto warmed fruit in dessert cups, top with sprinkled Cocoa mixture

Per serving, 110 calories

• • •

Lemon Mousse with Fudge Sauce

4 oz non-fat sugar-free yogurt
1 tsp artificial sweetener
1 teaspoon Sugar-free Lemon Jello
optional: 1/4 cup sliced strawberries, 3 walnut halves

Stir the sweetner & Sugar-free lemon Jello into yogurt. Mix well & spoon into dessert cups. Per serving, 60 calories; topped with 2 tablespoons of fudge sauce, 100 calories

Lime & Chocolate Dazzler

4 oz non-fat sugar-free yogurt
1 tsp artificial sweetener
1 teaspoon Sugar-free Lime Jello
2 tbsp Chocolate Sauce
1 or 2 strawberries, sliced

Mix artificial sweetener & Lime Jello into yogurt; spoon into dessert cup. Arrange strawberries over the lime, then top with Chocolate Sauce. Decadent-looking, but only **110** calories!

• • •

Cheesecake

pkg. Knox unflavored gelatin
2/3 cup boiling water
ice cubes
8 oz. Fat Free Cream Cheese ....210 calories in whole container
2 tsp vanilla extract
2 cups cold fat-free milk
Jell-o Sugar-Free Fat-Free Cheesecake mix, 1 pkg---280 c. in Cheesecake mix including milk, divided by 8 = 61 calories per serving.

Make crust first, directions below. While crust cools, dissolve gelatin into boiling water, stir until dissolved. Add 4 or 5 ice cubes, stir until mixture starts to thicken, remove ice cubes.
At medium speed blend cream cheese, vanilla extract, & 1/2 cup of the milk.
Then add rest of the milk & the Cheesecake mix; whisk until mixture thickens. Fold in the semi-thickened gelatin. Pour into pie plate, refrigerate for 4 hours. Top with drizzled fudge sauce & fruit if desired.

Serves 8, **61** calories per serving. If you add (25 cal.) 1/4 cup sliced strawberries or blueberries, it's **86** calories. Garnish with 2 tbsp (40 cal.) fudge sauce = **126** cal. per serving

Healthy pie crust

Makes 8 servings
1 cup quick oats .... 300 calories
1/4 cup oat or whole wheat flour .... 75 calories
1/2 cup Splenda
1/4 tsp salt
1/2 cup Diet Sprite
1 tbsp canola .... 120 calories
Mix canola with 4 tbsp warm water. With a fork beat until frothy, then add to crust mix.

Preheat oven to 400°. Spray 9" pie dish with cooking spray. In a bowl mix the oats, flour, Splenda, & salt. Add diet soda, mix; then add frothed canola/water. Press crust into plate bottom, moistening fingertips if needed.

Bake at 400° for about 12 minutes. Crust is **62** calories per serving

126 + 62 = **188** calories per cheesecake serving (with fruit & fudge topping)

PART THREE
A Physician Explains Tests, Drugs, & Doctor-Speak

If you do not change direction, you may end up
where you are heading. - Lao Tzu

Before Joyce continues with recipes, I should go over some tests and terms with you. Maybe you've just been to your doctor's office, and he's tried to explain things like your C-RP, HbA1c, Triglycerides, IFG, BUN & Creatinine findings.

Whew. If you were a NASA scientist it would make your head spin – plus it's hard concentrating on anything when you're feeling anxious, fearful of what it all means. I'd be terrified.

So first, wonderful news: **Your body is miraculous. It just needs a little help from you.**

In the U.S., the 40% of yearly deaths (not to mention illness) due to heart disease, stroke, and diabetes are *preventable.* How? *Just lose the weight.* It should be so simple. Remember Tom Hanks's character in CASTAWAY? Pudgy & out of shape at the beginning, lean & muscular at the end. How did he "do it?" (The Dieter's Refrain.) He spent months washed ashore on a desert island. He had no choice but to *move,* struggle physically, catch fish with a spear, collect wood for his fire, build his raft to sail for home.

He had to transform himself physically and emotionally to survive.

Imagine how you would survive, on a desert island with no junk food; no apparent food at all unless you work for it, move, be anything but sedentary.

Remember the "Amazing Facts About Your Heart and Blood Sugar" on page 17? I'll go over them again:

1. Your blood sugar starts dropping with the first pound you lose. In fact, with just the first *ounces* off, you've made yourself healthier. (Overweight is also a huge risk factor for breast and ovarian cancer in women, prostate cancer in men, and colon cancer in both men and women.)

2. Your heart, which is the size of your closed fist, is a small, overworked muscle, pumping 24/7. *And for every extra pound of fat you carry, your body has to grow seven new miles of blood vessels*; work that much harder. Put on two pounds and that's fourteen new miles of blood vessels; fifty extra pounds requires 350 miles of new blood vessels.

But the opposite is true. For every pound of fat you lose, your body sheds seven miles of blood vessels. They just re-absorb, break down, and get excreted. Lose two pounds and that's fourteen miles of blood vessels gone, lightening your heart's load.

So let these words be your mantra: **EVEN A LITTLE IS A LOT.**

Now I'll run through tests like the following, and their meanings.
1. Total Cholesterol
2. LDL
3. HDL
4. Triglycerides
5. Glucose
6. FBS & IFG
7. HbA1c
8. C-RP
9. BUN & Creatinine

1. <u>**Total Cholesterol**</u> means the sum of your LDL plus your HDL plus one-fifth of your Triglycerides (see #4).

2. <u>**LDL**</u> means low density lipoproteins; the lower the better. The optimal values for LDL have been adjusted downward several times in the last few years. Below 100 is the current target for people with no or few risk factors, below 70 for people with multiple risk factors. LDL provides the transport for cholesterol to reach and gum up your arteries. Anti-oxidants partially disable LDL. Saturated fats and trans-fats raise it; polyunsaturated and monounsaturated fats lower it.

3. <u>**HDL**</u>: high density lipoproteins, the higher the better. HDL is best over 40-45 in males, 50 in females. It has the opposite function to LDL. It transports cholesterol to the liver to be disposed of. It is more difficult to raise HDL than to lower LDL. Exercise and low carbohydrate intake will increase your HDL. Both HDL and LDL can be favorably influenced by a number of drugs, particularly the statin drug group.

4. <u>**Triglycerides**</u> are your basic fatty molecules. Your triglyceride number should be as low as possible, and rises with increased carbohydrate intake.

5. <u>**Glucose**</u> is your blood sugar number. The normal range is roughly 70-100. Your blood sugar varies a lot depending on how long ago you ate & what you ate. There are two main tests to evaluate it: the FBS & the HbA1c. (see below.)

6. <u>**FBS**</u> means fasting blood sugar, your glucose level (or number) after not eating for eight hours, usually overnight. If your FBS number falls between 100-125, that's called <u>**IFG**</u>, which means impaired fasting glucose, or pre-diabetes. Over 125 means diabetes.

7. The <u>**HbA1c**</u> (also called glycosylated hemoglobin, or glycohemoglobin) is a blood specimen test, whose readout will map your average blood sugar number during the past two to three months. The normal number is 5.0-6.0. From 6.0 to 7.0 corresponds to pre-diabetes. Above 7.0, serious diabetic complications often ensue.

8. The <u>**C-RP**</u> is a measure of the <u>inflammation</u> of your

coronary arteries' inner lining. Inflammation contributes to atherosclerosis[17], the laying down of cholesterol inside the arteries. Slowly, steadily, this narrowing of your arteries suffocates your heart muscle and brain for oxygen-carrying blood, raising the danger of heart attack and stroke.

9. <u>BUN</u> and <u>**Creatinine**</u> are blood tests to measure possible kidney failure, a serious diabetic complication and part of the Metabolic Syndrome.

Hope these explanations help. Especially since most of those test results come in the mail. You're alone, probably feeling alarmed, confused, holding a two-page printout of unintelligible terms and numbers. You run to call the doctor to find out -- and in these get-'em-in-get-'em-out HMO days, wait...and...wait, and finally (more often than not) get a call back not from the doctor but from a hurried nurse or clerk. Still more questions? It's right there! In your printout! Click.

No wonder people fear trips to the doctor.

Atherosclerosis means cholesterol depositing inside your arteries, slowly narrowing them, choking the heart and brain for oxygen-carrying blood. *It is caused by eating.* Decrease the wrong fats and carbohydrates. Eat anti-oxidants to prevent injury to your artery walls & decrease your arteries' inflammation. Your insulin sensitivity will also improve (the ability of your body to use up the sugar circulating in your blood.)

The Hierarchy of Bad Fats:

Most terrible: Trans fats, that commercial invention of man whose dangers you didn't know about for 15 years. Trans fats are/were the most atherosclerotic. They are metabolic poison.

Second worst: Saturated fats, less atherosclerotic than trans fats;

17   The word atherosclerosis comes from "athero" -- Greek for porridge. Picture warm, yellow, gooey gunk.

more atherosclerotic than cholesterol.

Least bad of the bad: Cholesterol, still atherosclerotic. Don't drive yourself crazy counting every mg.; just roughly remember: 300 mg. of cholesterol is the maximum safe daily amount for people with NO cardiovascular risk factors. For people with one or two cardiovascular risk factors the maximum is 200 mg; and for people with three or more risk factors, the maximum amount is 100 mg. The body also makes its own cholesterol.

Red meats, dairy products, skinless chicken, fish, and shellfish all contain the same amount of cholesterol (about 70 mg. per 4 oz serving). BUT red meats and dairy products are also high in saturated fat, whereas chicken, fish, & shellfish aren't. You don't want both cholesterol *and* saturated fat.

Important Medications: While this book is about weight loss, the ultimate purpose is your good health. And sometimes, despite good diet and exercise, you may also need medications to achieve this. Your Internist or Cardiologist may advise medication, usually after an initial several months of diet and exercise.

For **Cholesterol**, the main medications are the statin drugs, such as Lipitor (atorvastatin), Crestor (rosuvastatin), simvastatin, etc. The statins act mainly in the liver to favorably alter LDL/HDL production. They also benefit the inner lining of the artery wall (the endothelium).

Other drugs which act in a variety of ways are Ezetimibe, Niacin in high dose, Colestid, etc. These all have side effects, and need to be monitored by a physician. A new drug not yet approved in the U.S. as of this writing is rimonabant (Acomplia, Zimulti), a Sanofi-Aventis compound which is specific for the metabolic syndrome, causing weight loss and improvement in the cholesterol and diabetes profile, thereby reducing atherosclerosis.

For **Blood Pressure**[18], drugs have been available for 50 years. The most commonly used today are diuretics, beta-blockers, calcium channel blockers, ACE inhibitors and Angiotension Receptor Blockers. These too need to be prescribed by and monitored by a physician.

For **Diabetics**, there are numerous drugs, such as a variety of short and long acting Insulin compounds, and oral drugs such as metformin and the thiazolidinedione [glitazone] group.

Daily **aspirin**, if recommended by your doctor, has an anti-clotting effect, and has been shown to reduce the incidence of coronary events.

Vitamins: There is no objection to the typical one per day multivitamin. Re: minerals -- you get enough of them in a reasonable diet. Watch out for vitamins containing Iron, it can accumulate in the body and cause damage to liver, pancreas and heart. Use on your doctor's recommendation.

Need it still be said? **Tobacco** in any form will negate most of your other health-seeking efforts. For decades it's well established that smoking causes or contributes to lung cancer, esophageal cancer, bladder cancer, etc., plus it is one of the three major risk factors, along with cholesterol and high blood pressure, in causing heart attack and sudden cardiac death.

A friend was at her wit's end trying to get her son, influenced by peers, to stop smoking. Finally she burst out, "Honey, *it's just not cool to be stupid!*"

It worked. Well done, Mom.

---

18   Cardiovascular risk begins to increase above a blood pressure of 120/80. Drugs like diuretics, alpha- and beta-blockers, calcium channel blockers, ACE (angiotensin converting enzyme) inhibitors and ARB's (angiotensin receptor blockers) can also lower blood pressure in addition to weight loss and sodium restriction in the diet.

Diet Drugs: Most physicians are unenthusiastic about diet drugs. The patient learns nothing from such drugs, and quickly regains lost weight after the (unsustainable) drug is stopped. Plus there are the side effects, some just nasty, others lethal.

Available now are orlistat (side effect: oily diarrhea and soiling), and silbutramine (an amphetamine derivative, which can raise pulse and blood pressure). Other drugs have been removed from the market because of lethal damage to heart valves.

Mood:

We all have stress, but some people turn especially to food for comfort when feeling tense, angry, or depressed. Sometimes it's hard to know if depression was partly a cause of obesity, or if the obesity provoked the depression. Both should be recognized and treated. The hardest thing is understanding that your emotions can be your worst enemy. Stress from family, the job, other pain and frustration...*try to hang on, keep yourself together.* In your worst moments remember: THERE'S ONLY ONE PERSON IN THIS WORLD WHO CAN HURT YOU, AND THAT'S YOU.

Diets that "don't work:"

1. Short term or crash diets, often bizarre and failing to provide basic essential nutrients. 2. Diets you can't live with contentedly for the rest of your life. 3. Group dieting programs requiring weigh-ins and pep talks: most people drop out because of the time commitment, cost, or boredom.
4. Prepared meals served to your door: very expensive.

Confusion from the blizzard of misinformation:

Skepticism is good for you, especially when someone wants to sell you something. Reading/hearing about a product on TV or online, in magazines and books, doesn't always make it so. Eye critically the extravagant claims of celebrities, aerobics gurus, chefs at swanky restaurants, salesmen masquerading as experts, and yes, even M.D.s who lack *lifelong internal medicine experience* caring for patients, trying to prevent the suffering caused by overweight and obesity.

Advice coming from, say, the Mayo Clinic, would never ask you for money.

Deception in the stores: "No trans fats!" read the labels now -- but what have they replaced it with? Check especially Nutrition Facts labels of margarine, so-called diet foods, and pre-packaged frozen meals. See the *saturated fat*? In fine print: "1.5g saturated fat per serving." C'mon. If it's margarine, who eats just one teaspoon? And if the package says, No Cholesterol! Made with soy or canola oil!...have they *hydrogenated* those otherwise good oils? Sneeea-ky. You could hydrogenate extra virgin olive oil & it would still become...trans fat! Avoid even "partially hydrogenated" products.

Another deception lately is not listing how much sugar's in the product: it's hidden in the general term "carbohydrates." Sneeea-ky.

Summing up: Foods with 40 or 50 grams of carbs per serving don't tell you on the pretty package front that that includes 20 grams of sugar. Plus, what matters is the *kind* of fat and carbs you eat -- that's why they hide the sugar & saturated fat.

Shield children from the incessant advertising of junk food, the fast food places everywhere. Just say, "It's bad for you, honey. They just want to make money. Bet they don't let their own kids eat that stuff." And if peers drag your child into McDonald's or some such, just tell him or her to order salad, no dressing, & the leanest chicken possible, if they have it.

Before You Begin Your Diet: Start with a periodic complete physical at a time interval appropriate for your age and health, adding certain tests as you get older: Blood pressure, cholesterol, sugar, Pap smear, mammography, PSA in males for prostate evaluation, screening for colon cancer, etc. Add to this proper weight, good diet, exercise, no tobacco, and you have the makings of a healthy lifestyle. Work you like helps, other interests, and a stable social network.

The Body Mass Index [BMI]:

Ahead, the Table, but first some background info. The normal BMI is 18.5 – 24.9. Overweight is 25.0-29.9; Obesity is 30.0 and over. There is a formula for calculating the BMI from your height and weight, which uses the metric system. If you're mathematically inclined (Joyce isn't), the BMI means Weight in kilograms divided by the Height in meters squared. (She just hollered.) So okay, it's also Weight in pounds divided by Height in inches squared, then multiplied by the conversion factor of 703 (she just tossed a pillow at me).

On the next page you'll find the BMI chart. On the left find your height, then move across the line until you find your weight. The number above the intersection of those two will give you your BMI.

BMI														
	19	20	21	22	23	24	25	26	27	28	29	30	35	40
Height (in.)								**Weight (lb.)**						
4'10"	91	96	100	105	110	115	119	124	129	134	138	143	167	191
4'11"	94	99	104	109	114	119	124	128	133	138	143	148	173	198
5'0"	97	102	107	112	118	123	128	133	138	143	148	153	179	204
5'1"	100	106	111	116	122	127	132	137	143	148	153	158	185	211
5'2"	104	109	115	120	126	131	136	142	147	153	158	164	191	218
5'3"	107	113	118	124	130	135	141	146	152	158	163	169	197	225
5'4"	110	116	122	128	134	140	145	151	157	163	169	174	204	232
5'5"	114	120	126	132	138	144	150	156	162	168	174	180	210	240
5'6"	118	124	130	136	142	148	155	161	167	173	179	186	216	247
5'7"	121	127	134	140	146	153	159	166	172	178	185	191	223	255
5'8"	125	131	138	144	151	158	164	171	177	184	190	197	230	262
5'9"	128	135	142	149	155	162	169	176	182	189	196	203	236	270
5'10"	132	139	146	153	160	167	174	181	188	195	202	207	243	278
5'11"	136	143	150	157	165	172	179	186	193	200	208	215	250	280
6'0"	140	147	154	162	169	177	184	191	199	206	213	221	258	294
6'1"	144	151	159	166	174	182	189	197	204	212	219	227	265	302
6'2"	148	155	163	171	179	186	194	202	210	218	225	233	272	311
6'3"	152	160	168	176	184	192	200	208	216	224	232	240	279	319
6'4"	156	164	172	180	189	197	205	213	221	230	238	246	287	328

Body Mass Index according to height and weight.

Adapted from the National Institutes of Health Tables.

I do hear people ask, What's so bad about Overweight (BMI 25-30) or Obesity (BMI over 30)?

Answer: It's a living hell sentence of being sick, otherwise known as the **Metabolic Syndrome**: Central Obesity, High Blood Pressure, High Cholesterol and Triglycerides, High Blood Sugar (Diabetes), and Cardiovascular Disease: (angina, heart attack, heart failure, stroke, kidney failure, peripheral arterial disease, amputation).

In addition – I must say it again -- overweight is a definite risk factor for breast and ovarian cancer in women, prostate cancer in men, and colon cancer in both men and women. Getting sick, then sicker, & then desperately ill -- that is the fear. For many, more than dying.

To use the Body Mass Index Table below (**BMI**), find your height in the left-hand column. Look across the row for the weight closest to yours. The number at the top of the column is the BMI for your height and weight.

Do you want to dodge the bullet?

Consider everything I've just said as that image: THE BULLET.

You have not just split seconds, as in war, but months and maybe years to *transform yourself physically and emotionally.*

Heart attacks & strokes don't just happen, they are not in our stars, perhaps a little in our genes, but mostly in our refrigerators and overstocked pantries.

We've been perfecting this diet for 30 years, using the *selective* fat and carb principles we've described. But this sudden, great boon of new food products has us hugely excited, and Joyce has learned how to integrate them into our regular diet. *Finally*, in response to belated government pressure, food manufacturers have created and marketed delicious new foods of no or very low sugar, trans fat, and saturated fat. Oh joy. HEY WORLD, IT'S EASIER & FUNNER THAN EVER TO LOSE WEIGHT! BE HEALTHY! START SECOND OR THIRD CAREERS AT AGE 60, 70, OR 80…instead of…well, visit a ward of sick people, with the tubes & monitors & motorized chairs & trouble walking & breathing. WHICH do you want? Choose one, devote yourself to it with the focus and tenacity of a marine…and it's yours.

Now, more recipes. And a surprise: from here on Joyce will do it differently. She'll print each recipe twice. On each left page, she'll show you the old way, the old ingredients, underlining the villains to replace. And on the right, she'll show you *how to replace the villains* with healthy ingredients.

So consider each recipe a lesson too, teaching the bigger picture of how to replace and substitute in everything you eat, cook, and bake. Soon you'll be doing it automatically. Even thinking of the bad old stuff will make you shudder…yes, that will happen!

Good luck losing the weight.

Be happy.

PART FOUR

Hidden Sugar In Your Old Diet Recipes

It's gonna take a lot of fireworks to clean this place up.
-Homer Simpson

The usual game: if the recipe says it's fat-free, it's crammed with sugar. If it's sugar-free, it's loaded with fat...which metabolizes from sugar anyway if there's too much in the diet ...so let's concentrate on sugar in its "innocent" disguises.

Consider this casserole recipe for diabetics & obesity sufferers: "Replace sugar with one 12-ounce can (1 1/2 cups) of evaporated fat-free milk. Sound healthy? *Not.* One of those cans contains 300 calories and 45 g carbs -- which equal 11 tsp sugar. That's a candy bar! For someone already ill, it's poison. For someone just trying to lose weight, it's deception. Another gimmick is listing just "Carbs" on the recipe or food product label – instead of admitting that there's 35 grams of sugar per serving. And if that "serving" is tiny, who's going to eat just one?

There's more deception (brown sugar is sugar!), but fruits are up there too. Dates[19], so frequently substituted for sugar, are the most sugar-crammed fruit. Next come raisins & any dried fruit, but there are also crammed-with-sugar "sugar substitutes" like <u>honey, molasses, & maple syrup</u>. Per cup, honey has 1031 calories and 278 grams of Total Sugars, which equals 70 teaspoons of sugar! Want me to continue? They're all just sugar in colored liquid solution, no different from the sugar in your sugar bowl.

Below is a list of **Sugars in Disguise**. Adapt it to your needs.

19   See note, bottom p. 6

Understand that, besides nice flavor & fiber, they're all just sugar by another name. If you're only trying to lose weight, just go by calorie count. If you're pre-diabetic or diabetic, factor it in; be aware. In either case, realize that those dates, raisins, or brown sugar can be replaced by low cal ingredients in this diet's recipes to come.

FRUIT	CALORIES Per cup	TOTAL SUGARS
*Apple Sauce (unsweetened)	100	25 g
Apple Sauce (regular)	200	42 g
Apples (dried, diced)	210	50 g
*Apricots(dried, diced)	315	70 g
Banana, mashed	200	28 g
Blueberries (fresh)	83	14 g
*Blueberries (dried)	520	128 g
*Cranberries, dried	370	26 g
Currants, fresh	63	8 g
*Currants, dried	407	97 g
*Dates (dried, pitted)	501	113 g
Pineapple, fresh, diced	80	16 g
Pineapple, canned, drained	109	26 g
*Raisins	500	98 g

Avoid too **All-purpose flour**. It's in nearly every diet recipe, on nearly every diet site. Why? Because it makes things taste better (& the Diet popular). Its outer husk was removed to make foods lighter & fluffier, but that whole-grain husk, with its slow enzymatic breakdown, was what gave slower sugar absorption; avoided the glucose/insulin highs and crashes. All-purpose flour metabolizes almost as fast as sugar -- & with 456 calories per cup, of which 95 grams of carbs quickly convert into *24 teaspoons of sugar*[20]. Better to stick to whole grain flours. I'll teach you how to cook & bake with whole wheat pastry flour, soy flour, & milled flaxseed -- which, with its heart-healthy Omega-3 oils, helps to reduce the risk of heart disease, lowers cholesterol, and helps to fight cancer.

Beware too of "diet" recipes telling you to use: **butter**, stiff with saturated fat. Since trans fats are out, Diets & Diet magazines are suddenly extolling the "old time natural goodness of butter." Sure, it's gloriously delicious but...die another day. Diet recipes also tell you to use **cake flour, corn muffin mix,** etc. Don't. You know what's in them.

Ahead are sample teaching recipes, each taking up two pages. On the left pages, I'll show you current Diets' villain ingredients. And on the right I'll show you how to replace them with new, healthy products. Also *add* because you *can*; these new substitutions are both delicious and low-cal. Soon you'll be doing this automatically[21], replacing and substituting in everything you eat, cook, and bake. Improvise. Get creative!

But don't go overboard. Remember that even whole grains, while better for you, have carbs which metabolize into sugar, and plenty of calories too.

---

20   Every 4 g of carbs = 1 tsp sugar. Divide Total Carbs by 4.

21   Don't drive yourself crazy counting carbs. Just have a rough idea & be aware.

Replace with New Food Products & Cooking Techniques: a few examples, unhealthy ones on the Left.

<u>Shrimp Tetrazzini</u> Found this -- ack -- in a magazine for diabetics & pre-diabetics. The hidden sugars in it are killers. Recipe says it "Makes about 6 *small** servings, 215 calories each." And: "5 g Total Fat, 1 g sat. fat...? 24 mg chol, 35 g carbs." Does that sound right? Take a look; do the math.

Cooking spray
4 oz dried whole wheat spaghetti Not a bad start but: 400 cal, 86 g carbs = *22 teaspoons sugar metabolized*) (*divide Total Carbs by 4 to get # tsp sugar*)
<u>1/2 cup all purpose flour</u> ....228 cal, 48 g carbs = *twelve tsp sugar*
<u>1 12 ounce can (1 1/2 cups) evaporated fat-free milk</u> ...300 cal, 45 g carbs = *11 teaspoons sugar*)
1 12/ cups sliced mushrooms
1 cup chopped red & green peppers
1/2 cup cold water (for mixing the unnecessary flour)
1/8 tsp salt
1/8 tsp black pepper
1 cup frozen pre-cooked shrimp...................................... 100 cal
<u>1/2 cup shredded Parmesan cheese</u> ....216 cal, 2 g carbs
3 tablespoons fresh parsley

Cook spaghetti according to package directions. Drain. In large skillet lightly sautee the mushrooms & pepper. Stir the flour into the cold water. Pour flour mixture into the vegetable mixture in the skillet. Stir in evaporated milk, salt, & pepper. Stir until thickened. Stir in the cooked spaghetti, shrimp, Parmesan cheese, and parsley. Etc.

*Those "6 servings" are tiny. 1cup shrimp & 4 oz spaghetti for 6 people? More likely this would serve 4, at 324 calories each, with tons of sugar.

Shrimp Tetrazzini

Serves 4, at 121 calories per serving, with bigger, more filling portions of shrimp and fat free cheese. To make it even healthier broccoli, which is rich in vitamins C & A, has as much calcium as a glass of milk, and potent cancer-fighting components, has been added.

Cooking spray
8 oz TofuShirataki noodles (per 2 oz serving:10 calories, 3 g carbs, 0 fat, 0 cholesterol) .... 40 cal
1/2 cup chopped onions .... 30 cal
1 cup sliced mushrooms .... 15 cal
1/2 cup chopped red peppers .... 30 cal.
2 tbsp dried garlic
fresh ground black pepper to taste
1 tbsp dried parsley
1 1/2 cups frozen pre-cooked shrimp .... 150 calories
1 cup broccoli florets, frozen ok .... 40 cal
1 cup shredded Fat Free cheese .... 180 calories

Preheat over to 350. Spray skillet & baking dish with cooking spray. In the skillet sautee onions, mushrooms, & peppers, sprinkling with garlic, pepper & parsley. Add shrimp & broccoli last; simmer.

Rinse noodles well & microwave for a minute. Drain noodles, leaving a little water in them. Mix cheese into still-hot noodles. Then fold in the whole shrimp and vegetable mixture, tossing as cheese melts.
Spoon shrimp-noodle mixture into baking dish. Cover & bake for 15 minutes. Cool 5 minutes before cutting and serving.

Tofu Shirataki noodles are available either from house-foods.com, Amazon.com (gourmet), Trader Joe's, and health stores.

Lemon Couscous Chicken

This recipe is popular in North Africa. It's also found in major Diets. The problem here is couscous, another of those good-for-you misconceptions. It's just another flour with its husk removed. (proof: how fast it fluffs up). 1 pkg of Couscous mix contains 220 calories & 40 g carbs which equal 10 g sugar, into which it quickly metabolizes like white flour or rice.

Cooking spray
1 1/2 pounds skinned chicken breast
salt & pepper to taste (avoid salt: it retains water & raises blood pressure)
1 small onion, sliced thin
1 1/4 cup water
1 tsp paprika
1 1/2 tsp cinnamon
1 pkg Couscous mix
Juice of 1 lemon
1/4 tsp lemon peel

Cut chicken and season with salt and pepper. In a skillet cook chicken until golden. Reduce heat. Add onion to pan and cook until softened. Add paprika & cinnamon, stir. Add water and contents of the spice sack from the couscous mix. Bring to a boil, stir in the couscous and lemon. Remove from heat, cover, let stand for 5 minutes. Fluff with a fork.

Serves 6
Per Serving: 290 cal, 40* g carb, 8 g fat, 1 g sat. fat, 70 mg chol

40 carbs will quickly metabolize into 10 teaspoons of sugar. Would you eat 10 teaspoons of sugar from the sugar bowl?

MLA Lemon-Soy Chicken

Soy flour thickens like flour but *isn't* flour; it comes from legumes (beans). 1/4 cup has 120 calories, 8 g Total Carbs, 3 g dietary fiber, 2 g sugar, and *huge amounts of protein.* 1/4 cup soy flour = 1 hamburg or 4 oz chicken.

Cooking spray
1 1/2 pounds skinned chicken breast
fresh ground pepper to taste
1 small onion, sliced thin
2 tsp garlic
2 tsp cinnamon
1 1/2 tsp ginger
2 cups broccoli florets (frozen ok)
1 cup chicken broth
<u>1/4 cup soy flour</u>
2 tablespoons Splenda
juice of 1 lemon & 1 tsp lemon peel
1/2 cup slivered almonds---Like walnuts, a daily handful of almonds has heart-healthy, cholesterol-lowering and weight maintenance capabilities.

Spray skillet with cooking spray. Cut chicken into smaller pieces, season with fresh ground pepper. Over medium high heat, cook chicken on both sides until golden. *Pour off drippings,* and reduce heat.
Add onion to pan and cook until softened. Add garlic, cinnamon, ginger & broccoli. Stir.
To the chicken broth add soy flour & Splenda, microwave for one minute, stir, pour into chicken mixture; stir again. Add almonds, lemon juice, & lemon peel.
Remove from heat & serve hot

Serves 6. Per Serving: 177 cal, 1.7 g carb, 1 g. unsaturated fat, 70 mg chol

If you miss the couscous, try this with **Cauliflower Crunchies,** p. 142. You may even like them for snacking!

Pizza

This Major Diet "pizza" has too many calories for something so tiny.

1 7" round pita
1/4 cup bottled pizza sauce
1/3 cup chopped veggies (onions, mushrooms, etc.)
pepper to taste
1/4 cup crumbled part-skim mozzarella*

Preheat oven to 400. On a baking sheet spread pizza sauce over the pita.
Sprinkle the cheese over the pizza sauce and top with veggies.
Bake in oven for 5 minutes or until cheese is melted.

Per serving: **236** calories, 29 g carbs, 7 g fat, 3 g saturated fat, 17 mg cholesterol, 4 g fiber

*In 1/4 cup (100 calories), part skim mozzarella still has 4 g saturated fat & 20 mg cholesterol. Why not just have a cookie?

Pizza

Nutrient-packed & way more filling.

Whole Wheat & Soy Flour Crust:
Cooking spray
1 pkg. Active dry yeast
1 cup water (warm)
4 tbsp Splenda
1 1/2 cup Whole Wheat Pastry Flour
1/2 cup Soy Flour---1/2 cup soy flour has 2 g saturated fat, 0 mg.
cholesterol, & 20 g of protein -- as much as in two hamburgers.

Spray large bowl and pizza pan with cooking spray. Sprinkle yeast
into water, stir & let stand until "creamy," about 10 minutes. Add
Splenda, then both flours & work to form dough. Place in lightly
oiled bowl. Cover & let rise about 45 minutes. Punch down &
spread on lightly oiled pizza pan.

Tomato Sauce: 1/2 cup to spread on pizza dough. **80** calories

Topping:
Cooking spray
1/2 cup sliced onions
1/2 cup sliced mushrooms
1/2 cup crumbled Fat Free Mozarella---*No Fat* Mozarella: 84
calories per *1/2* cup, Total Fat 0, cholesterol 10 mg., Total Carbs 0,
Dietary Fiber 1 g

Preheat oven to 400 degrees. Spray pizza pan with cooking spray.
Put dough onto a surface lightly floured with soy flour & roll into a
ball. Flatten into a circle & transfer to lightly oiled pizza pan. Place
floured fingertips in center; press & push outward toward edges,
rotating pan as you go, making the crust almost thin. When dough
reaches edges, spread with Tomato Sauce. Sprinkle mozzarella onto
sauce & top with veggies. Bake *on lowest shelf* for 15-20 minutes or
until golden brown. Let cool slightly before cutting.

Serves 6. each serving, **190** calories, sat fat **.3** g, cholesterol 3 mg.,
Total Carbs 19 g, Dietary Fiber 9 g

Reduced Fat Mayonnaise

Looked up the ingredients, let's see...20 calories per serving (1 level tbsp), Total Carbs 2 g, Total Fat, 2 g, Saturated Fat 0 g, Poly- & Monounsaturated Fat 1 g, Trans Fat 0 g....*waitamminit.* It doesn't add up! If the Total Fats are **2 g,** & the good poly-& mono-unsaturated fats only equal 1 g -- *where's the missing gram?* SEE P. 46, or let me quote from that page:

"The FDA guidelines instituted on January 1, 2006 have been a disappointment, because food manufacturers can actually claim that their product is trans fat-free <u>as long as it contains less than 1/2 gram (500 mg.) per serving</u>[22]. <u>Worse, THEY decide what a serving size is, and it's ridiculously tiny.</u> You would consider a serving size as three times what they do, but this labeling loophole has allowed trans fats back into the stores and your home. "That's extremely disturbing," said Michael D. Ozner, M.D., chairman of the American Heart Association of Miami, "since as few as three daily servings of these supposedly safe foods can increase one's risk of heart disease and diabetes by thirty percent."

"Heart Healthy! 0 trans fat!" says one brand of cracker. But what *is* their "serving?" Two little crackers? And if those two crackers add up to 499 mg., *which makes it legal to say they have no trans fat* -- and meanwhile you're happily chowin' 'em down because you think it's ok...where does that leave you?" Back to unknowingly harming yourself..."

As for that REDUCED FAT MAYONNAISE. That 0 next to their Trans Fat? That could be 499 mg, 1 mg shy of 500...which makes it LEGAL for them to say 0 trans fat. Meanwhile you're scooping & spreading the stuff on your rollup or salad, thinking it's ok, it's healthy.

You've just overdosed on trans fats. According to the USDA[23], over 42,000 food products on the market still contain trans fats, including forty percent of all prepared foods such as margarines,

---

22   Cf. Pgs. 46-47

23   January, 2007

baking mixes, desserts, spreads, chips, crackers, granola bars, cereals, and frozen foods.

• • •

Mayonnaise Healthy Substitute

Mix these three together & put on your salad or rollup. You'll swear it's mayonnaise!

1/2 cup non-fat plain or Greek yogurt .... 50 calories
1/2 tsp powder of Sugar-Free Jello Vanilla pudding .... 5 c.
1/2 tsp powder of Sugar-Free Jello Lemon gelatin .... 5 c.

Tuna Salad: Serves 2; 167 calories per serving

1 can Solid White Albacore Tuna (in water, drained) 225 calories
1 cup chopped onions, celery & tomatoes .... 50 c.
1/2 cup plain non-fat yogurt .... 50 c.
1/2 tsp Sugar-Free Jello Vanilla pudding .... 5 c.
1/2 tsp Sugar-Free Jello Lemon gelatin .... 5 c.

Mix together the two Jello products & the yogurt. Add in the tuna, onion, celery & tomatoes; arrange on lettuce -- or between 2 slices healthy bread *because you can*, you've saved so many calories.

We all love corn but it too becomes sugar…and seems to be on nearly every diet site. Do people feel it's an acceptable substitute for flour? It isn't. Corn, potatoes, rice & white flour all break down rapidly to sugar (a bit slower than table sugar but still fast) & cause your insulin to spike, which makes you hungry again too fast.

1. Spicy Chicken with <u>Corn</u> Relish
4 skinned chicken breast halves
1/2 tsp chili powder
1/2 tsp salt
Green & red peppers, diced
1 small onion, diced
1 olive oil-flavored vegetable cooking spray
<u>1 16-ounce package corn</u>---55 g carbs, which equal almost 14 tsp sugar

2. <u>Corn</u> Casserole
8-oz. can <u>creamed corn</u>---yow.
<u>canned whole kernel corn</u>
<u>sugar</u>, 2 tsp
egg substitute---not much help.
<u>6-1/2 oz. pkg corn bread mix</u>---see below.
canola or corn oil

3. Corn Bread Mix   Advertised as low in cholesterol & gluten-free, but its Percent of *Calories from Fat is 17 %, & from Carbs 91 %.* Then most packages say, way at the bottom, "Total may exceed 100% due to rounding," whatever that means. Corn Bread Mix is also high in added sugar (before the corn itself is metabolized), & contains preservatives.

A pity. Corn is comfort food and people yearn for that – or at least for something yummy & seemingly starchy to go with, say, chicken or turkey.

So try the **Crunchies** -- with turkey? -- on the facing page. You may be surprised.
Turkey Breast

Bake a big, fresh turkey breast. Line pan with heavy-duty aluminum foil for easy clean-up. Follow directions on wrapping except: peel off every bit of skin & fat. Use scissors to snip as you go. Brush lightly with oil & cover with foil tent. Re-baste once during cooking. In the last 20 minutes remove foil so surface will turn golden, re-basting again if necessary.

Note: Even de-skinned & de-fatted, you'll be amazed at how much juice (liquid fat) pools in the pan. Use the baster tube to suction some out. Careful: it's hot.

When done, let cool a bit & slice away...for days. Sandwiches, salads, casseroles, & snacks. Cooking big poultry is easy. Who needs the deli?

• • •

Cauliflower Crunchies:

Preheat oven to 400. Fresh or frozen cauliflower is ok. Just let the frozen thaw a bit, & if you want the pieces smaller, cut them.

Line a wide pan with aluminum foil, then spray it with cooking spray. Into a plastic bag put soy flour & pepper to taste. (Soy flour is 100 calories per 1/4 cup, mostly protein.) Shake the bag in your hands to mix the soy and pepper.

Now load in the cauliflower, half the amount at a time, and shake the bag to cover thoroughly. Arranged "breaded" Crunchies on the lightly oiled pan. Spray their tops with cooking spray.

Bake in hot oven for 5 minutes or until golden brown.

Quiche

This, from 2 Major Diets (recipes nearly identical)

<u>8 eggs</u> . . . . = 2,400 mg cholesterol.
(ga-a!)
1 cup skim milk
<u>3/4 cup shredded Swiss cheese</u> . . . . = 130 mg cholesterol
1 10 oz pkg frozen broccoli
1 teaspoon salt---retains water; raises blood pressure
1/4 teaspoon pepper
1/4 teaspoon ground nutmeg
1/4 teaspoon pepper
<u>3 tablespoons shredded Parmesan cheese</u> . . . . . .12 mg cholesterol
<u>12 oz. cooked crisp turkey bacon crumbled</u>. . .312 mg. cholesterol
(googled: manufacturer describes 1/2 oz as a serving, so *12 oz
equals. . .24 servings*)

Heat oven to 350. Spray 9" pie plate with Pam; set aside. Mix eggs
& skim milk in a lg. bowl. Fold in cheese, spices & turkey bacon.
Pour into greased pie plate and bake for 50 minutes until golden
brown, or until knife inserted in center comes out clean. Serve
immediately.

2,854 mg of cholesterol. That's insane. Not even worth counting
the calories.

MLA Quiche

This is so low in calories & cholesterol you can have crust too. Make the crust first, in fact. Quiche like this is great for lunch, dinner, anytime.

Healthy pie crust: Makes 1 for a 9 inch pie, 6 servings
1 cup quick oats ....300 calories
1/4 cup oat or whole wheat flour......75 calories
1/2 cup Splenda
1/2 cup Diet Sprite
1 tbsp canola ..120 calories---Mix canola with Sprite. Beat with a fork until frothy, then add to crust mix.

Preheat oven to 400°. Spray 9" pie dish with cooking spray. In a bowl mix the oats, flour, & Splenda. Add diet soda, mix; then add frothed canola/water. Press crust into plate bottom, moistening fingertips if needed.
82 calories per serving

Quiche, Serves 6

Cooking spray
1 cup sliced onions & mushrooms ....50 calories
1 1/2 cups Liquid Egg Whites (12 oz.) ....200 "
1 cup shredded fat free cheddar cheese................180 "
1 cup broccoli ....25 "
1 tsp salt, 1/2 tsp pepper, 1 tsp ground nutmeg

Spray skillet with cooking spray. Sautee onions & mushrooms; add broccoli & stir briefly. Into pan pour the eggs, cheese, & spices, stirring until cheese melts & mixture looks soupy. Pour into crust and bake for 15-20 minutes, or until knife inserted in center comes out clean. Serve immediately.

*Quiche without crust: 76 calories per serving.
*Quiche with crust: 158 calories per serving; equals 2 tsp sugar from metabolized oats & wheat flour

Chocolate Chip Cookies

Still a popular "diet" recipe, no different from non-diet recipes except for the Splenda. Big deal.

<u>1 cup all-purpose flour</u>: No way this amount of flour can produce 36 cookies, unless they're the size of bottle caps. And who eats just 1 or 2?
1/2 tsp baking soda
1/4 tsp salt
<u>1/2 cup butter:</u> Butter is saturated animal fat. Since trans fats are "out," Diets are back to combining saturated fat with less than 1/2 g. trans fat per tiny "serving." But you'll use more than 1 "serving." See p. 46, underlined text.
<u>1 egg:</u> in one yolk, 300 mg. cholesterol.
1 tsp vanilla extract
1/3 cup Splenda
<u>2/3 cup firmly packed brown sugar:</u> 553 calories, 141 grams Total Sugars
<u>1/2 cup semi-sweet chocolate chips:</u> *Eeyew*: 640 calories, 80 g Total Carbs, 20 g sugar, 32 g Total Fat, Saturated Fat, 20 grams

Yield: 36 (?) servings. Says the recipe, "Calories 75, Total Fat 3g, Saturated Fat 1g, Cholestrol 15 mg, Total Carbohydrate 10 g, Sugars 7g."

Okay, let's say their numbers are correct & someone eats *only 3* of these tiny cookies. That's **225** calories, Total Fat 9 grams, Saturated Fat 3 grams, Cholesterol 45 mg, Total Carbs 30 grams, Sugar 21 grams....

...I count more, but let's skip that and kick out those unhealthy calories. Double the *SIZE* of the cookies & replace them with super-healthy (and more filling) ingredients.

Chocolate HEALTHY Cookies Delicious too.

As fun as junk food but contain more nutrients than most meals.

Cooking spray
1 cup quick oats .... 300 cal, 54 Total Carbs, Diet Fiber 8 g
1/4 c whole wheat flour...110 cal, 23 Total Carbs, Diet Fiber 4 g
1/2 cup Splenda
1/4 cup chopped walnuts .... 192 calories
1/4 cup dried blueberries .... 140 calories
1 1/2 tablespoons baking powder
1 teaspoon baking soda
2 tbsp canola .... 240 calories
4 tbsp warm water
1 teaspoon vanilla extract
1/2 cup chocolate sauce

Preheat your oven to 400°. Spray cookie pans with cooking spray. In a bowl combine the oats, flour, Splenda, walnuts, blueberries, baking powder & baking soda. With a fork, spend 2-3 minutes "frothing up" the oil and water. Add the chocolate sauce & vanilla extract to the oil & water mixture, & combine with the dry ingredients.

Drop batter by rounded tablespoonfuls onto pans, flatten slightly with fingers, & bake for 10 minutes. Cool 2-3 minutes, then move to cookie racks.

Yield: 10 cookies, 114 calories each

Natural Unsweetened Cocoa powder has eleven times more antioxidants than blueberries and 29 times more antioxidants than broccoli. It also has the most antioxidants of chocolate products (followed distantly by dark chocolate — which, *avoid when combined with saturated fat and sugar.*)

Apple Muffins

As any cook knows, Splenda alone in baking doesn't work; you have to replace half with sugar if you want to "make the cookie stiff."

<u>1 3/4 cups all purpose flour</u>
<u>1/2 cup sugar</u> ("divide by half with Splenda")
2 tsp baking powder
1/2 tsp baking soda
1/2 tsp salt
<u>1 egg</u>, beaten (1 yolk alone contains 300 mg. cholesterol)
1 1/2 cups chopped apples
3 tbsp canola
1/2 cup skim milk
1/2 cup chopped walnuts

Preheat oven to 400. Spray muffin cups with Pam

Blend dry ingredients in a bowl. In a separate bowl, combine egg, oil, & milk. Add dry ingredients to egg mixture; stir until blended. Fold in apples & nuts. Batter will be thick.

Fill well-greased muffin cups 2/3 full. Bake at 400 for 18-20 minutes or until top springs back when touched.

Servings: 12

Apple Muffins

Cooking spray
3/4 cup Whole Wheat Pastry Flour
3/4 cup quick cook oatmeal
3/4 cup Splenda
2 tsp baking powder
1/2 tsp salt
1 1/2 tsp Ener-G Egg Replacer + 3 tbsp warm water
3 tbsp canola
1 1/2 cups unsweetened applesauce
1/2 cup skim milk
1/2 cup chopped walnuts
more Splenda

Preheat oven to 400. Spray 12 muffin cups with cooking spray.

Blend dry ingredients in a bowl. In a separate measuring cup, mix the egg replacer & warm water; then add canola & fork-whisk all three until frothy. Set aside for a sec.
Quickly add applesauce, milk, & nuts to dry ingredients; stir. (Optional: save some of the nuts to sprinkle on unbaked muffins.) Add canola/egg replacer/water froth last, & stir again.

Fill muffin cups 2/3 full. Sprinkle tops with chopped nuts & more Splenda. Bake at 400 for 18-20 minutes or until top springs back when touched.

Servings: 12, **130** calories each, Total carbs 10, Dietary carbs 4.2

In addition to spices, a standard pumpkin pie recipe calls for more than 3/4 cup white sugar, 2 –3 egg yolks, and 1 12-oz can of evaporated milk. That's hugely fattening – one 12-oz can of innocent-sounding fat free evaporated milk has 45 g carbs, which quickly break down to 11 tsp sugar. Then there's the lardy, sugary, floury pie shell.

Try this no sugar, fat or cholesterol **HEALTHY PUMPKIN PIE** recipe.

Serves 8 at **112 calories** per serving, including the crust. (Make the crust first.)

3/4 cup Splenda
1/2 tsp salt
1 tsp cinnamon
1/2 tsp ground ginger
1 can pumpkin filling .... 140 calories
*1/2 cup liquid egg whites .... 67 c.
*1/4 cup fat free shredded mozzarella cheese .... 45 c.
4 tsp egg replacer .... 40 c.
6 tbsp warm water

Preheat oven to 400 degrees. Combine the first four ingredients in a small bowl. Stir pumpkin into skillet & heat slowly. Add the egg whites and fat free cheese, stirring until cheese starts to melt. (If the eggs start to cook, remove from heat for a bit.) Stir in the Splenda and spice mix. Mix egg replacer well with water, add, stir whole mixture, pour into crust.

Bake at 400 degrees for 10 minutes. Reduce temperature to 350, bake 15-20 more minutes or until toothpick inserted comes out clean.

The cheese is what "binds." Blended with the egg whites, the two substitute beautifully for the innocent-sounding, not-healthy evaporated milk. (Fat free, nice, but as much sugar as a candy bar.) And you needn't bake at such high temps for so long, because you're not waiting for sugar to melt, egg yolks to cook – and you've already heated your ingredients. Experiment with the cheese/egg whites ratio. 12 oz liquid is what you need (8 oz egg whites & 4 oz melted cheese), though you may want to put a bit more cheese in. The bland white kind doesn't affect the pie's wonderful flavors.

Index

A

Anytime Blondies, p. 92
Anytime Brownies, p. 94
Anytime Cheese & Onions Bar, p. 96
Anytime Cheese & Turkey Bar, p. 97
Apple Crisp, p. 125
Apple muffins, p. 169
Artificial Sweeteners, p. 26
Atherosclerosis, p. 140

B

Berry Intense Smoothie, p. 98
Black Cherry Chocolate Mousse, p. 132
Banana muffins, p. 90
Blondie, p. 92
Brownie Anytime, p. 94
Brownie, New Age p. 129

C

Cappuccino p. 127
Cardiologists, p. 18-19
Cauliflower Crunchies, p. 142
Central Obesity, p. 28

Cheesecake, p. 133

Cheese 'n Onions Bar, p. 96

Cheese '& Turkey Bar, p. 97

Cheese and Veggies Pita Pocket, p. 91

Chicken Cacciatore p. 110

Chicken, Lemon Soy, p. 136

Chicken Marsala, p. 102

Chicken Parmigiana, p. 120

Chicken Penne Rigate with Mushrooms & Broccoli, p. 108

Chicken, Polynesian p. 102

Chicken Stroganoff, p. 117

Chicken Tarragon with grapes & walnuts, p. 111

Chicken Tex Mex, p. 88

Chilli, p. 116

Chocolate Berry Parfait p. 123

Chocolate Blueberry Bits, p. 150

Chocolate Blondies, p. 82

Chocolate Candy, p. 131

Chocolate Cookies, p. 167

Chocolate drink, p. 88

Chocolate Frosting, p. 149

Chocolate ice cream, P. 126

Chocolate Mousse, p 128

Chocolate pudding with strawberries p.127

Chocolate sauce, p. 122

Chocolate Smoothie, p. 98

Chicken Tarragon with grapes & walnuts, p. 111

Cocoa, p. 88

Cookies, Chocolate, p. 149

Crunchies, p. 142

Crunchy Fruit rollup, p. 90

Crudites, p. 106

Crust, Healthy, p. 165

D

E

Eggs, Scrambled & cheese pita, p. 99

F

"Fat gene," p. 24

Fettucini Alfredo, p. 104

Flaxseed, milled, p. 20 (note)

Frosting, p. 130

Fructose, danger p. 25

Fruit Chocolate Fondue p. 126

Fruit Rollup, p. 84

Fudge Frosting, p. 130

Fudge Nut Tart p 124

Fudge Sauce, P. 122

G

Garlic shrimp & Vegetables p. 114

Gout, p. 28

H

Harvard School of Public Health, p. 9

HDL, p. 29

Henry VIII, p. 28

Hot cocoa, p. 88

I

Ice Cream, Chocolate, Vanilla etc. p. 126

J

K

L

Lasagna p. 118

Latte, Mocha p. 99

LDL, p. 29

Lemon-garlic Marinated Shrimp p. 107
Lemon Mousse p. 132
Lemon-Soy Chicken, p. 136
Lime & Chocolate Dazzler p. 133
Linguine with White Clam Sauce p. 112

M
Mayonnaise, "Reduced" fat p. 160
Mayonnaise, healthy substitute p. 161
Meatballs, Fat free ground turkey, p. 113
Metabolism, p.15
Mini-quiches, p. 100
Mocha Latte, p. 99
Mousse, Orange Walnut with Fudge Sauce p. 112
Mousse, Chocolate p. 128
Mousse, Lemon p. 117
Muffins, Apple p. 148
Muffins, banana, p. 90

N
New Age Brownie, p. 117
New Healthy Food Products, p. 51
Nova Scotia omelet, p. 112

O
Omelet, western, p. 107
ORACs, p. 112, p.151
Orange Walnut Mousse with Fudge Sauce p 123

P
Pancake, New Age, p. 89
Pancake, Pita, p. 87
Pear, Pudding & Chocolate Sauce, p. 124
Penne Rigate with Chicken& Broccoli, p 121
Phlebitis, p. 28
Pie crust, p. 144 & p. 152

Pita, Cheese & Veggies Pita Pocket, p. 80
Pita Pancake, p. 87
Pita, Tomato & Cheese, p. 91
Pita, Scrambled eggs & cheese, p. 99
Pizza, p. 138
Polynesian Chicken p. 115
Popcorn, p. 71
Pumpkin Pie, p. 170

Q
Quiche, p. 165
Quiches, mini, p. 100

R
"Reduced" Fat Mayonnaise, p. 141
Rye & Cheese Sandwich, p. 99

S
Salmon Dijon, p. 105
Scrambled eggs & cheese pita, p. 99
Shrimp, Lemon-garlic marinated p. 107
Shrimp Scampi p. 119
Shrimp Tetrazzini, p. 134
Shrimp with Vegetables p. 101
Smoothie, Berry Intense, p. 98
Smoothie, Chocolate p. 98
Smoothie, Strawberry, p. 98
Soy Protein Powder, p. 83
Spaghetti & *MLA meatballs, p. 113
Stevia, p. 27
Stir-Fry vegetables, p. 108
Sugar Alcohols, p. 25
Sweeteners, Artificial, p. 26

T
Tex Mex Chicken, p. 103

Tomato sauce, p. 113
Tomato & cheese Pita, p. 91
Top Antioxidants Table, p. 150
Trans fats in our food, pgs 51-52 & 160
Tuna Melt Rollup, p. 101
Tuna Salad p. 161
Tuna Vinaigrette, p. 109
(Vinaigrette sauce, p. 106)
Turkey & Cheese Bar, p.97
Turkey rollup, p. 100

U

V

Vanilla ice cream, p. 126
Vanilla pudding, p. 126
Vinaigrette, p. 106

W

Western Omelet, p. 107

X

Y

Z